Medical Glossaries in the Hebrew Tradition: Shem Tov Ben Isaac, *Sefer Almansur*

Études sur le Judaïsme Médiéval

TOME LXXII

The titles published in this series are listed at *brill.com/ejm*

Medical Glossaries in the Hebrew Tradition: Shem Tov Ben Isaac, *Sefer Almansur*

With a Supplement on the Romance and Latin Terminology

By

Gerrit Bos
Guido Mensching
Julia Zwink

BRILL

LEIDEN | BOSTON

Library of Congress Cataloging-in-Publication Data

Names: Shem Tov ben Isaak, of Tortosa, active 13th century, author. | Bos, Gerrit, 1948- writer of added text. | Mensching, Guido, writer of added text. | Zwink, Julia, writer of added text. | Shem Tov ben Isaak, of Tortosa, active 13th century Sefer Almansur. | Shem Tov ben Isaak, of Tortosa, active 13th century Sefer Almansur English. | Rāzī, Abū Bakr Muḥammad ibn Zakarīyā, 865?–925? Kitāb al-Manṣūrī.
Title: Medical glossaries in the Hebrew tradition : Shem Tov ben Isaac, Sefer Almansur : with a supplement on the Romance and Latin terminology / by Gerrit Bos, Guido Mensching, Julia Zwink.
Other titles: 880–01 Sefer Almansur.
Description: Leiden ; Boston : Brill, [2017] | Series: Études sur le Judaïsme médiéval ; 72 | Includes indexes. | Text in English and Hebrew, with some footnotes containing Arabic terms.
Identifiers: LCCN 2017028041 (print) | LCCN 2017029224 (ebook) | ISBN 9789004352032 (E-book) | ISBN 9789004352025 (hardback : alk. paper)
Subjects: LCSH: Medicine, Medieval–Terminology. | Medicine, Arab. | Hebrew language, Medieval–Glossaries, vocabularies, etc. | Arabic language–Transliteration into Hebrew. | Latin language, Medieval and modern–Transliteration into Hebrew. | Shem Tov ben Isaak, of Tortosa. Sefer Almansur.
Classification: LCC R128.3 (ebook) | LCC R128.3 .S5413 2017 (print) | DDC 610.1/4–dc23
LC record available at https://lccn.loc.gov/2017028041

Typeface for the Latin, Greek, and Cyrillic scripts: "Brill". See and download: brill.com/brill-typeface.

ISSN 0169-815X
ISBN 978-90-04-35202-5 (hardback)
ISBN 978-90-04-35203-2 (e-book)

This book is printed on acid-free paper and produced in a sustainable manner.

Contents

Preface

The current publication is an edition, translation, and study of the Arabic–Romance list of medicinal ingredients (pharmacopeia) with a concise description of their properties in terms of hot or cold and their therapeutical uses, as it features in the *Sefer Almansur* by Shem Tov ben Isaac of Tortosa. The book is a continuation and addition to the study of the medical terminology featuring in this list that was published recently.[1] The Romance (mostly Old Occitan) and Latin terminology, which is partially identical to that of Shem Tov ben Isaac's *Sefer ha-Shimmush*,[2] is studied in the supplement at the end of this volume.

Our studies of the *Sefer Almansur* have been highly stimulated by several projects funded by the Deutsche Forschungsgemeinschaft (DFG), whom we would like to thank. In particular, our work on the Supplement on the Romance and Latin terminology is part of the DFG-funded project, "An XML-based Information System for Old Occitan Medical Terminology". Finally, the authors thank the anonymous reviewers for their useful comments and suggestions for corrections.

---

1 Gerrit Bos, "Shem Tov Ben Isaac, *Sefer Almansur*," in *Novel Medical and General Hebrew Terminology from the 13th Century*, vol. 2, = *JSS*, Supplement 30 (2013): 1–20.

2 Gerrit Bos, Martina Hussein, Guido Mensching, and Frank Savelsberg (eds.), *Medical Synonym Lists from Medieval Provence: Shem Tov Ben Isaac of Tortosa, Sefer ha-Shimmush, Book 29. Part 1: Edition and Commentary of List 1 (Hebrew–Arabic–Romance/Latin)* (Leiden: Brill, 2011); Gerrit Bos, Fabian Käs, Jessica Kley, Guido Mensching, and Frank Savelsberg (eds.), *Medical Synonym Lists from Medieval Provence: Shem Tov Ben Isaac of Tortosa, Sefer ha-Shimmush, Book 29. Part 2: Edition and Commentary of List 2 (Romance/Latin–Hebrew–Arabic)* (forthcoming).

Sigla and Abbreviations

א Ms Vatican, Urbinati hebr. 50: fols. 41b–48b
ב Ms Jerusalem, The National Library of Israel, Heb. 4⁰1099: fols. 18b–22b
O Ms Oxford, Bodleian Library 592, Marsh 376: fols. 72a–80b

AdOr Raymond Arveiller. *Addenda au* FEW XIX *(Orientalia)*, ed. Max Pfister. Tübingen: Niemeyer, 1999.

AdV Arnaldi de Villanova. *Translatio libri Albuzale De medicinis simplicibus*, eds. José Martínez Gázquez and Michael R. McVaugh = *Arnaldi de Villanova Opera medica omnia*, vol. 17. Barcelona: Publicacions i Edicions de la Universitat de Barcelona, 2004.

BDB Francis Brown, Samuel R. Driver, and Charles A. Briggs. *A Hebrew and English Lexicon of the Old Testament: With an Appendix containing the Biblical Aramaic, based on the Lexicon of William Gesenius as translated by Edward Robinson*. 1907, repr. Oxford: Oxford University Press, 1978.

BKM Gerrit Bos, Dorothea Köhler, and Guido Mensching. "Un glosario médico-botánico bilíngüe (iberorromance-árabe) en un manuscrito hebráico del siglo XV." In *Actas del* IX *Congreso Internacional de Historia de la Lengua Española (Cádiz, 2012)*. Vol. 2, ed. José María García Martín, 1763–1776. Madrid: Iberoamericana-Vervuert, 2015.

BM Eliezer Ben Yehuda. *Millon ha-Lashon ha-Ivrit: Thesaurus Totius Hebraitatis et Veteris et Recentioris*. 17 vols. 1910–1959, repr. Tel Aviv, 1948–1959.

DAO Kurt Baldinger, ed. *Dictionnaire onomasiologique de l'ancien occitan*. Tübingen: Niemeyer, 1975–.

D Reinhart P.A. Dozy. *Supplément aux Dictionnaires arabes*. 2 vols. Leiden: Brill, 1927.

DCVB Antoni M. Alcover and Francesc de B. Moll. *Diccionari català-valencià-balear*. 2nd ed. 10 vols. Palma de Mallorca: Moll, 1980–1985.

DECLC Joan Coromines. *Diccionari etimològic i complementari de la llengua catalana*. 10 vols. Barcelona: Curial / Fundació Coromines-Ara Llibres, 1980–1991.

DETEMA María Teresa Herrera. *Diccionario español de textos médicos antiguos*. 2 vols. Madrid: Arco Libros, 1996.

DT Albert Dietrich, ed. and trans. *Dioscurides Triumphans: Ein anonymer arabischer Kommentar (Ende 12. Jahr. n. Chr.) zur Materia medica. Arabischer Text nebst kommentierter deutscher Übersetzung*. 2 vols. = Abh. der Akad. der Wiss. in Göttingen, Phil.-Hist. Klasse, Dritte Folge, vol. 172. Göttingen: Vandenhoeck & Ruprecht, 1988.

DW Max Wellmann, ed. *Pedanii Dioscuridis, Anazarbei De Materia Medica Libri Quinque*. 5 bks. in 3 vols. Repr., 1 vol. Berlin: Weidmann, 1958.

FAB Jehuda Feliks. *Animals of the Bible and Talmud*, in: *Encyclopaedia Judaica*, vol. 3, pp. 7–19.

FAQ Irene Fellmann. *Das Aqrābādīn al-Qalānisī. Quellenkritische und begriffsanalytische Untersuchung zur arabisch-pharmazeutischen Literatur*. Beirut: Steiner, 1986.

FEW Walther von Wartburg. *Französisches Etymologisches Wörterbuch*. 25 vols. Bonn, Leipzig, Tübingen, Basel, 1922–1987.

GGA Alejandro García González, ed. *Alphita: Edición crítica y comentario*. Firenze: Sismel, 2007.

GH Karl Ernst Georges. *Ausführliches lateinisch-deutsches Handwörterbuch*. 2 vols. 1913–1919, repr. Darmstadt: Wissenschaftliche Buchgesellschaft, 1995.

HebMedSyn Gerrit Bos and Guido Mensching. "The Literature of Hebrew Medical Synonyms: Romance and Latin Terms and their Identification," *Aleph* 5 (2005): 169–211.

IB Ibn al-Bayṭār. *al-Jāmiʿ li-mufradāt al-adwiya wa l-aghdhiya*. 4 pts. in 2 vols. Beirut, 1992.

IBF Ibn al-Bayṭār, *Traité des simples*, trans. Lucien Leclerc. 3 vols. Paris: Impr. nationale, 1877–1883.

ID Aḥmed Issa. *Dictionnaire des noms des plantes en latin, français, anglais et arabe*. Cairo, 1930.

IĞ Ibn Ǧanāḥ. *Kitāb al-Talḫīṣ*, ed. and trans. Gerrit Bos and Fabian Käs (forthcoming).

IT Gerrit Bos, Guido Mensching, and Julia Zwink. *Commentary on the Romance and Latin Terms in Moses Ibn Tibbon, Sefer Ẓedat ha-Derakhim, bk. 7. chs. 7–30* (forthcoming).

JD Marcus Jastrow. *A Dictionary of the Targumim, the Talmud Bavli and Yerushalmi, and the Midrashic Literature*. Repr., 2 vols. New York: Pardes, 1950.

KB Ludwig Koehler and Walter Baumgartner. *The Hebrew and Aramaic Lexicon of the Old Testament: Subsequently revised by W. Baumgartner and J.J. Stamm, with assistance from B. Hartmann, Z. Ben-Hayyim, E.Y. Kutscher, Ph. Reymond, translated and edited under the supervision of M.E.J. Richardson*. 5 vols. Leiden: Brill, 1994–2000.

KM Fabian Käs. *Die Mineralien in der arabischen Pharmakognosie: Eine Konkordanz zur mineralischen Materia medica der klassischen arabischen Heilmittelkunde nebst überlieferungsgeschichtlichen Studien* = Akademie der Wissenschaften und der Literatur Mainz. Veröffentlichungen der Orientalischen Kommission, vol. 54. 2 vols. Wiesbaden: Harrasowitz, 2010.

L — Edward W. Lane. *Arabic-English Lexicon.* 8 vols. London: Williams and Norgate, 1863–1879.

LF — Immanuel Löw. *Die Flora der Juden.* 4 vols. 1928–1934, repr. Hildesheim: Olms, 1967.

Low — Adolph Lowinger. "Register of Hebrew and Aramaic terms, translated and edited by S. Paley." In *Biblisch-talmudische Medizin: Beiträge zur Geschichte der Heilkunde und der Kultur überhaupt*, by Julius Preuss. Repr., New York, 1971.

LR — François J.M. Raynouard. *Lexique roman: Ou dictionnaire de la langue des troubadours comparée avec les autres langues de l'Europe latine.* 6 vols. 1838–1844, repr. Heidelberg: Winter, 1970.

LS — Henry G. Liddell and Robert Scott. *A Greek–English Lexicon. Revised and augmented throughout by H.S. Jones* a.o. With a supplement 1968, repr. Oxford: Clarendon, 1989.

M — Max Meyerhof, ed. *Maimonides, Sharḥ asmāʾ al-ʿuqqār, un glossaire de matière médicale composé par Maïmonide.* 1940, repr. in *Islamic Medicine*, vol. 63, ed. Fuat Sezgin. Frankfurt am Main: Institut für Geschichte der Arabisch-Islamischen Wissenschaften, 1996; Engl. trans.: Fred Rosner, *Moses Maimonides' Glossary of Drug Names: Translated and annotated from Max Meyerhof's French edition* = Maimonides' Medical Writings 7. Haifa, 1995.

MA — Moses Maimonides. *Medical Aphorisms. Critical editions of the Hebrew translations by Nathan ha-Meʾati and Zeraḥyah Ben Isaac Ben Sheʾaltiel Ḥen*, ed. Gerrit Bos (forthcoming).

MBG — Gerrit Bos and Guido Mensching. "A Medico-Botanical Glossary in Hebrew Characters of Italian Origin." *Iberia Judaica* 6 (2014): 11–21.

MLWB — Paul Lehmann. *Mittellateinisches Wörterbuch bis zum ausgehenden 13. Jahrhundert.* Vol. 1: A–B; vol. 2: C. Munich: C.H. Beck, 1967–1999.

NM 1 — Gerrit Bos. *Novel Medical and General Hebrew Terminology from the 13th Century: Translations by Hillel Ben Samuel of Verona, Moses Ben Samuel Ibn Tibbon, Shem Tov Ben Isaac of Tortosa, and Zeraḥyah Ben Isaac Ben Sheʾaltiel Ḥen* = JSS, Supplement 27 (2011).

NM 2 — Gerrit Bos. *Novel Medical and General Hebrew Terminology from the 13th Century, Volume Two.* = JSS, Supplement 30 (2013).

NM 3 — Gerrit Bos. *Novel Medical and General Hebrew Terminology, Volume Three: Hippocrates' Aphorisms in the Hebrew Tradition* = JSS, Supplement 37 (2016).

NM 4 — Gerrit Bos. *Novel Medical and General Hebrew Terminology, Volume Four* (forthcoming).

NPRA	Jacques André. *Les noms de plantes dans la Rome antique*. Paris: Les Belles Lettres, 1985.
PSW	Emil Levy. *Provenzalisches Supplement-Wörterbuch: Berichtigungen und Ergänzungen zu Raynouards Lexique roman*. 8 vols. Leipzig: Reisland, 1894–1924.
RMA	Clovis Brunel. "Recettes médicales d'Avignon en ancien provençal." *Romania* 80 (1959): 145–190.
SC	Francis Steingass. *A comprehensive Persian-English Dictionary*. 1892, repr. 1984.
SDA	Michael Sokoloff. *A Dictionary of Jewish Babylonian Aramaic of the Talmudic and Geonic Periods*. Ramat Gan: Bar Ilan University Press, 2002.
SHS 1	*Medical Synonym Lists from Medieval Provence: Shem Tov Ben Isaac of Tortosa, Sefer ha-Shimmush, Book 29. Part 1: Edition and Commentary of List 1 (Hebrew–Arabic–Romance/Latin)*, eds. Gerrit Bos, Martina Hussein, Guido Mensching, and Frank Savelsberg. Leiden: Brill, 2011.
SHS 2	*Medical Synonym Lists from Medieval Provence: Shem Tov Ben Isaac of Tortosa, Sefer ha-Shimmush, Book 29. Part 2: Edition and Commentary of List 2 (Romance/Latin–Hebrew–Arabic)*, eds. Gerrit Bos, Fabian Käs, Jessica Kley, Guido Mensching, and Frank Savelsberg (forthcoming).
Sin	Guido Mensching, ed. *La Sinonima delos nonbres delas medeçinas griegos e latynos e arauigos*. Madrid: Arco Libros, 1994.
SP	Werner Schmucker. *Die pflanzliche und mineralische Materia Medica im Firdaus al-ḥikma des ʿAlī ibn Sahl Rabban Ṭabarī*. Inaugural-Dissertation, Bonn, 1969.
ThLL	*Thesaurus linguae Latinae*. 10 vols. Stuttgart, Leipzig, 1900–.
UW	Manfred Ullmann. *Wörterbuch zu den griechisch-arabischen Übersetzungen des neunten Jahrhunderts*. Wiesbaden: Harrassowitz, 2002.
UWS	Manfred Ullmann. *Wörterbuch zu den griechisch-arabischen Übersetzungen des neunten Jahrhunderts. Supplement Band 1: A-O*. Wiesbaden: Harrassowitz, 2006.
WfP	Edward Larrabee Adams. *Word-Formation in Provençal*. New York: Macmillan, 1913.
WKAS	*Wörterbuch der klassischen arabischen Sprache*, ed. Deutsche Morgenländische Gesellschaft et al. Wiesbaden: Harrassowitz, 1957–.

Introduction

1 Multilingual Medical Glossaries in Hebrew Characters

In the various Christian realms on the Iberian Peninsula and in Southern France, Jewish doctors in the thirteenth and fourteenth centuries did not, like their Christian counterparts, have access to the medical schools, as for instance the one in Montpellier.[1] They received their basic medical training in a family setting, from father to son. The basic medical books used during these lessons were mainly medical works written in Arabic (composed in that language or translated from Greek): Hippocrates' works with Galen's commentaries, Alexandrian summaries, and the books by Ḥunayn b. Isḥāq, Ibn al-Jazzār, al-Zahrāwī, Ibn Sīnā, and others. In addition to these Arabic works, Hebrew translations may have played a role as well. Typically, however, they did not use Latin works or works composed in the vernacular. During this period, Jews and Christians did not live in a situation of "peaceful convivencia," but—as David Nirenberg has shown—"violence was a central and systemic aspect of the coexistence of majority and minority in medieval Spain."[2] He even suggests that "coexistence was in part predicated on such violence."[3] Time and again the Church and municipal authorities tried to discourage Christians from consulting Jewish doctors. Yet Jewish doctors were much in demand, not only by Jews but also by Christians, with their numbers testifying to their popularity: while constituting 3 to 5% of the total population in the major cities, their share in the medical profession was ten times that proportion.[4] Some restrictive measures were directed in particular against the acquisition of drugs from Jewish apothecaries in order to treat Christian patients. Thus, Pope Innocent IV issued a papal bull in 1250, which stated (among other things) that Christians might only use medicinal remedies that had been prepared by competent Christian apothecaries. The statutory code entitled "Las Siete

1 In the mid-fourteenth century, Jews could attend lectures in a medical faculty in Italy or Montpellier, but they could not take a degree; cf. Michael McVaugh, *Medicine Before the Plague: Practitioners and Their Patients in the Crown of Aragon 1285–1345* (Cambridge: Cambridge University Press, 1993), p. 100, n. 120.

2 David Nirenberg, *Communities of Violence: Persecution of Minorities in the Middle Ages* (Princeton: Princeton University Press, 1996), p. 9.

3 Ibid.

4 Joseph Shatzmiller, *Jews, Medicine, and Medieval Society* (Berkeley: University of California Press, 1994), p. 108.

Partidas," compiled during the reign of Alfonso x of Castile (d. 1284), forbade Christians from taking medicines prepared by a Jewish apothecary, though a Christian apothecary might prepare a drug for a Jewish doctor to administer.[5] In 1325 the council of Barcelona issued an ordinance that no Jew was to practice as an apothecary (nullus judeus ... uteretur officio apothecarie).[6] Although these measures were not always strictly observed, they did considerably limit the number of Jews having an apothecary.[7]

A consequence of such measures was that in order to treat his Christian patient, a Jewish doctor had to turn to a Christian apothecary to buy the drugs he needed for the patient, but in order to do that he had to know the Latin or vernacular name of the drug he wanted. The same was true if he bought the simple ingredients and prepared the drug himself, as some doctors did, or if in calling on a Christian patient in company with an apothecary he had to explain to his companion what medicine was required. The situation was further complicated if he moved to another region where a different language or dialect was spoken; this was the case of the Jewish doctor Shem Tov ben Isaac of Tortosa (where Catalan was spoken), who subsequently moved to Marseille (where people spoke Occitan). Yet many Jewish doctors were trained in Arabic–Hebrew medicine. They knew the Arabic names of the medicaments they needed for treating their Christian patients but often not the Latin and/or vernacular ones. In such cases they needed translations of the simple medicines prescribed by their medical handbooks. In order to fill this gap, Jewish doctors composed a large number of medical glossaries during the thirteenth to fifteenth centuries that correlated drug names in Arabic (Hebrew), Latin, and a Romance vernacular. Thus, these lists clearly served a practical purpose, and do not "embody a continued—albeit bookish—connection to Arab culture."[8] One of these doctors was Shem Tov ben Isaac of Tortosa.

5 McVaugh, *Medicine Before the Plague*, p. 59.

6 Ibid., p. 60, n. 87.

7 Shatzmiller, *Jews, Medicine, and Medieval Society*, p. 88, remarks that "Jews did not play any important part in pharmacy" and that "they are rarely seen as pharmacists, but when they are, they seem to be engaged in the profession in defiance of both the legislation and the custom of the land."

8 Cf. Paulina P. Lewicka and Gad Freudenthal, "The Reception and Practice of Rationalist Medicine and Thought in Medieval Jewish Comminities: East and West," in *The Routledge Handbook of Muslim–Jewish Relations*, ed. Joseph Meri (London: Routledge, 2016), p. 107. For the Arabic glossary tradition, cf. Peter E. Pormann and Emilie Savage-Smith, *Medieval Islamic Medicine* (Washington, DC: Georgetown University Press, 2007), p. 53: "These lists however, are not very consistent in their assignment of local terms, and much of the interest appears to have been antiquarian rather than practical."

2 Shem Tov Ben Isaac of Tortosa

Shem Tov ben Isaac was born in the Catalan city of Tortosa. He traveled to the Near East for business before, at the age of thirty, beginning to study in Barcelona at some point after under R. Isaac ben Meshullam. He subsequently spent some time in Montpellier, and was later active as a physician and translator in Marseille.[9] It was in the city of Marseille that Shem Tov translated al-Zahrāwī's *Kitāb al-taṣrīf*.[10] Calling it *Sefer ha-Shimmush*, Shem Tov started his translation in the year 1254 and completed it at an unknown date.[11] Next to the *Kitāb al-taṣrīf*, Shem Tov translated Abū Walīd Muḥammad Ibn Rushd's Middle

9 On Shem Tov ben Isaac, his life, and literary activity, see Ernest Renan, *Les Rabbins français du commencement du quartorzième siècle* (1877, repr. Farnborough: Gregg 1969), p. 592; Moritz Steinschneider, *Die hebräischen Übersetzungen des Mittelalters und die Juden als Dolmetscher* (1893, repr. Hildesheim: Olms, 1966), pp. 741–745; Heinrich Gross, *Gallia Judaica: Dictionnaire géographique de la France d'après les sources rabbiniques* (Paris: Cerf, 1897), pp. 375–376; Süssmann Muntner, "R. Shem Tov Ben Isaac of Tortosa about the Life of the European Jewish Doctor and His Ethics," in *Sinai Jubilee Volume*, ed. Yehuda Leib Maimon (Jerusalem: Mossad Harav Kook, 1957): 321–327; George Sarton, *Introduction to the History of Science*, vol. 2.2 (New York: Krieger, 1975), pp. 845–846; Shatzmiller, *Jews, Medicine, and Medieval Society*, pp. 44–45; Gerrit Bos, "The Creation and Innovation of Medieval Hebrew Medical Terminology: Shem Tov Ben Isaac, *Sefer ha-Shimmush*," in: *Islamic Thought in the Middle Ages: Studies in Text, Transmission and Translation, in Honour of Hans Daiber*, eds. Anna Akasoy and Wim Raven (Leiden: Brill, 2008): 197–202. This introduction is an adaptation of that which features in: Bos, Hussein, Mensching, and Savelsberg (eds.), *Medical Synonym Lists from Medieval Provence, Part 1*, pp. 10–11.

10 On the *Kitāb al-taṣrīf*, see Danielle Jacquart and Françoise Micheau, *La médecine arabe et l'occident mediéval* (Paris: Maisonneuve et Larose, 1990), pp. 139–141 and *passim*.

11 The year is derived from the introduction to the translation (cf. Muntner, "R. Shem Tov Ben Isaac of Tortosa", p. 325, § 5). In the same introduction, Shem Tov relates an incident that occurred in Marseille in the year 1261 (cf. Muntner, op. cit., p. 328, § 22). From this, it can be concluded that Shem Tov either wrote the introduction after compiling the lists and that the year 1261 marks its completion, or that he completed the work at an earlier date and then subsequently revised it, inserting the incident mentioned above in the process. The first assumption seems to be that of Moritz Steinschneider, *Die hebräischen Handschriften der K. Hof- und Staatsbibliothek in München*, 2nd rev. ed. (Munich: Palm, 1895), p. 2, no. 8: "Schemtob b. Isak (1254–61)." The second assumption seems to be that of Renan, *Rabbins français*, p. 592, who, however, draws on an unknown source to assert that Shem Tov completed the work in 1258 and then revised it in 1261. This is also the opinion of Sarton, *Introduction to the History of Science*, p. 846, and Shatzmiller, *Jews, Medicine, and Medieval Society*, p. 45. Steinschneider, *Hebräische Übersetzungen des Mittelalters*, p. 741, remarks that he completed the translation between 1261–1264 (= Muntner, "R. Shem Tov Ben Isaac of Tortosa," p. 322).

Commentary on Aristotle's *De Anima*,[12] Abū Bakr Muḥammad ibn Zakariyya al-Rāzī's medical compendium *K. al-Manṣūrī*,[13] and Hippocrates' *Aphorisms* with Palladius' commentary.

3 Shem Tov's Translation of the List of Medicinal Ingredients

In the original Arabic text of al-Rāzī's *K. al-Manṣūrī*, the list of medicinal ingredients figures at the end of book three[14] and bears the title "On remedies that are applied frequently." The Arabic list is arranged according to the *abǧad* alphabet and consists of the Arabic terms of the medicinal ingredients with a concise description of their properties in terms of hot or cold and their therapeutical uses. Thus it starts with

أسارون: حار ينفع من سدد الكبد ويدرّ البول جيّد للاستسقاء اللحمي.

> *Asārūn* is hot and good for an obstruction of the liver; it induces micturition and is beneficial for dropsy of the flesh.

In his translation of this list bearing the title "Chapter on the powers of the simple drugs which the physicians frequently used as part of their remedies and other [means of healing] at all times and arranged according to the alphabet" (שער בכחות הסמים הנפרדים אשר הרבו הרופאים להרגילם במרקחים וזולתם בכל העתים והם מסודרים על אלף בית), Shem Tov provides the reader not only with the original Arabic term, but in many cases also the Romance and in a few cases Hebrew equivalents. This list is thus different from the procedure adopted by him in

12 Cf. Steinschneider, *Hebräische Übersetzungen des Mittelalters*, p. 148; Averroes, *Middle Commentary on Aristotle's* De Anima: *A Critical Edition of the Arabic Text with English Translation, Notes, and Introduction*, ed. Alfred L. Ivry (Provo, UT: Brigham Young University Press, 2002), pp. xxviii–xxix and 150, n. 69.

13 Cf. Steinschneider, *Hebräische Übersetzungen des Mittelalters*, pp. 725–726. The *K. al-Manṣūrī*, dedicated by al-Rāzī in 903 to a local Iranian prince Abū Ṣāliḥ Manṣūr ben Isḥāq (which explains its popular title), governor of the town of Rayy near present-day Tehran, treats the whole medical theory and practice in ten books. Of the Latin translation made in Toledo during the twelfth century by Gerard of Cremona, the ninth book (Liber Nonus ad Almansorem), on therapeutics, was one of the most widely read medieval medical manuals in Europe, and it continued to be used as a university textbook well into the sixteenth century; cf. Pormann-Savage-Smith, *Medieval Islamic Medicine*, pp. 163–164.

14 For instance, in Ms Oxford, Bodleian Library, MS Marsh 376, it features on fols. 72ᵃ–80ᵇ.

his *Sefer ha-Shimmush*, i.e., his translation of al-Zahrāwī's *Kitāb al-taṣrīf*. In this translation Shem Tov replaced the original list of plants in Arabic, Greek, Syriac, and Persian with two lists. The first list consists of the Hebrew terms as they feature in his translation, alphabetically arranged, and their Arabic and Romance equivalents,[15] while the second list is an independent kind of vademecum starting in each entry with the Romance term, followed by its Hebrew and/or Arabic counterparts. The entries are alphabetically arranged.[16]

Shem Tov's *Sefer Almansur* is still extant in nine manuscripts; however, the list of medicinal ingredients can only be found in the following two:

1) Jerusalem, The National Library of Israel, Ms Heb. 4⁰1099; fols. 18^b–22^b; copied in the fourteenth century in a Sephardic semi-cursive script.[17] The manuscript suffers from occasional staining, which renders parts of the text illegible.
2) Vatican, Urbinati hebr. 50: fols. 41^b-48^b. The Ms consisting of 163 folios was copied in Spain or Provence in the first half of the fifteenth century in a Sephardic semi-cursive script.[18] The manuscript was owned by Menahem Volterra, whose signature appears on the first folio. At the top of the same page the estimated value of the manuscript, two florins, is marked נערך ב' פר. This seems to be the only complete copy of the translation extant and the only one with the translator's preface, in which Shem Tov devoted a chapter to the importance of acquiring knowledge of sciences in general and of medicine in particular. The manuscript ends with the following colophon on fol. 163a:

> נשלמת העתקת ספר אלמנצור בכל שעריו ומאמריו הנזכרים בתחלת הספר
> בחדש ניסן שנת חמשת אלפים ועשרים וארבע תהלה לאל עולם אשר אתו

15 For the edition of the first list, see Bos, Hussein, Mensching, and Savelsberg (eds.), *Medical Synonym Lists from Medieval Provence, Part 1*.

16 Cf. Shem Tov's statement (Bos, Hussein, Mensching, and Savelsberg (eds.), *Medical Synonym Lists from Medieval Provence, Part 1*, p. 16): "I have also composed an explanation of the drugs and herbs in the vernacular and Arabic so that someone who goes on a distant journey will know their names in both languages. And I have arranged them alphabetically." The edition of the second list by Bos, Kley, Mensching, and Savelsberg is forthcoming.

17 For the data regarding the Mss, see the *Online Catalogue of the Institute of Microfilmed Hebrew Manuscripts* at the National Library of Israel (hereafter IMHM), in addition to the catalogues mentioned with each entry. For the Jerusalem Ms, see also Rafael Weiser (ed.), *Sefarim mi-Sefarad* [*Books from Sefarad*] (Jerusalem: Ministry of Education and Culture, 1992), p. 130, no. 73. In our edition of terms this Ms is indicated by the siglum ב.

18 In our edition this Ms is indicated by the siglum א.

האמצע והעזר הסופר לא יזק לא היום ולא לעולם עד שיעלה חמור בסולם אשר
יעקב אבינו חלם ברוך הנותן לייעף כח ולאין אונים עצמה ירבה.[19]

This is the end of the translation of the *K. al-Manṣūrī* with all its books and chapters, which are mentioned in the beginning of the work. [I completed it] in the month of Nisan 5024 [= 1264], praise be to the everlasting God who has the means[20] to help. May the scribe come to no harm, not today and not ever, until a donkey climbs the ladder which Jacob our father dreamt. Blessed is He who gives strength to the weary, fresh vigor to the spent [Is. 40:29; trans. JPS].[21]

---

19 Cf. Steinschneider, *Hebräische Übersetzungen des Mittelalters*, p. 726; Benjamin Richler, *Hebrew Manuscripts in the Vatican Library: Catalogue. Compiled by the Staff of the Institute of Microfilmed Hebrew Manuscripts, Jewish National and University Library, Jerusalem. Palaeographical and Codicological Descriptions: Malachi Beit-Arié in collaboration with Nurit Pasternak* (Vatican City: Biblioteca Apostolica Vaticana, 2008), p. 632.

20 Lit., 'means and help.'

21 For the colophon, see Moritz Steinschneider, "Vorlesungen über die Kunde Hebräischer Handschriften deren Sammungen und Verzeichnisse: Mit einer Schrifttafel," *Centralblatt für Bibliothekswesen*, Beiheft 19 (1897): 48–49. The work has been reprinted in Amsterdam 1966 together with *Allgemeine Einleitung in die jüdische Literatur*, and *Zur pseudepigraphischen Literatur des Mittelalters*; Elkan Nathan Adler, "The Humours of Hebrew Mss.," in *About Hebrew Manuscripts* (1905, repr. New York: Sepher-Hermon Press, 1970), pp. 105–106; and especially Alexander Scheiber, "Donkey-ladder," *Folio Ethnographica* 1 (1949): 99–101, repr. in *Essays on Jewish Folklore and Comparative Literature* (Budapest: Akademiai Kiado, 1985): 19–22. According to Scheiber, the following concluding phrase "The end. May no harm befall the copyist until the donkey ascends the ladder, of which our father Jacob had dreamt" can be found frequently in Hebrew Mss kept in Germany, France, and Italy and even in a Hebrew Ms, which reached Hungary from Bohemia, as well as in later Hebrew printed works. Scheiber continues that "the general opinion has been that we have to deal here with an arbitrary metaphor of the copyists, expressive of impossibility, and meaning that the donkey was unable to ascend the ladder, so that no harm could befall the copyist." Its source can however, as Scheiber remarks, be found in an aggadic statement about the four impossibilities: "Four things were said by the wise: A sack can be washed white, so knowledge can be found with the ignorant; when the donkey ascends the ladder, then you can find wisdom with fools; when the kid puts up with the panther, then the daughter-in-law can put up with her mother-in-law; when you find an entirely white raven, then you find a good woman"; see also Benjamin Richler, *Hebrew Manuscripts: A Treasured Legacy* (Cleveland: Ofeq Institute, 1990), pp. 23–24. We thank Eric Pellow for this reference.

In addition to differences in physical condition and completeness, there is a significant discrepancy in the use of Romance terminology between the two surviving manuscripts. In the Vatican manuscript the Romance equivalents are unvocalized and fully integrated in the list. In contrast, in the Jerusalem manuscript, Shem Tov's Romance terminology is altogether lacking, and a copyist has supplied a variety of vowelized Romance and Latin equivalents in marginal glosses. However, because of the close correspondence between the Romance terminology used by Shem Tov in the *Sefer ha-Shimmush*[22] and the translation of the *K. al-Manṣūrī*, the Romance synonym terminology is, in our opinion, part of Shem Tov's original translation, and is the object of a detailed analysis and study in the supplement to this book.

As already mentioned in the preface, the particular Hebrew medical terminology has been studied on a previous occasion. The edition of the complete text of the glossary has once more confirmed the impression gained from this study, namely that in view of the relatively large number of novel terms—that is, terms that do not feature in the current secondary literature and dictionaries of the Hebrew language at all, or that do occur but in a different meaning—a proper understanding of this text in particular and of medieval medical literature in general is impossible without a proper inventory of these terms.[23] Some striking examples of such terms with novel, unattested meanings going back to the Arabic original term may substantiate our assertion. For instance, in Alef 9, Shem Tov uses the term שגעון not in the general meaning of "folly," but in that of "melancholy" (Arabic مالنخوليا); in Bet 2, Hebrew הקדיר does not have the general sense of "to darken," but of "to have a narcotic effect" (Arabic خدّر); in Bet 6, Hebrew הדרוקן does not mean "dropsy," but "colic," as Shem Tov generally uses the latter term for Arabic قولنج; in Bet 10, Hebrew נתק is not "scab," or "fungus," but "freckles" (Arabic كلف); in Zayin 9, Hebrew ילפת means "dandruff" (Arabic إبرية) and not the regular "scab(s)"; in Ḥet 4, Hebrew דשן (ashes) features in the sense of "ophthalmia" (Arabic رمد); in Ḥet 9, Hebrew הנעים (to make pleasant) has the meaning of "to fatten" (Arabic خصب); in Ṭet 4, the unattested Hebrew זיכום stands for "catarrh" (Arabic زكام); in Kaf 17 (and elsewhere), Hebrew לטישה (polishing) features in the sense of "cleansing" (Arabic جلاء); in Nun 4,

22 I.e., his translation of al-Zahrāwī's *Kitāb al-taṣrīf*.

23 For such inventories, cf. Gerrit Bos, *Novel Medical and General Hebrew Terminology from the 13th Century*, 2 vols, = JSS, Supplement 27, 30 (2011–2013); *Novel Medical and General Hebrew Terminology*, vol. 3: *Hippocrates' Aphorisms in the Hebrew Tradition*, = JSS, Supplement 37 (2016); and *Novel Medical and General Hebrew Terminology*, vol. 4 (forthcoming).

Hebrew חניקה (strangling) means "quinsy (angina)" (Arabic خوانيق); and in Qof 9, Hebrew טחורים (hemorrhoids) stands for Arabic بواسير in the sense of "(nasal) polyps."[24]

In light of its relative completeness and legibility, as well as the inclusion of Romance terminology typical of Shem Tov's work, this edition of the Arabic–Romance list is based primarily on the Vatican manuscript, with the exception of obvious scribal errors, in which case the Jerusalem manuscript has been consulted.[25]

The original Arabic text has been consulted throughout for variant readings and for those cases in which both Hebrew manuscripts have corrupt versions. The Arabic manuscript consulted is Oxford, Bodleian Library 592, Marsh 376 (folios 72^{a}–80^{b}), which was copied before 813/1410. It is an incomplete copy of the first five books of the *K. al-Manṣūrī*.[26]

4 Romance and Latin Terms

The list in the Vatican manuscript displays many entries containing Romance or Latin terms. These appear as "synonyms"[27] after the Arabic lemma, and before the Hebrew synonym (when present). These lexical equivalences are followed by a description of the respective substances or remedies, cf., e.g., entry Bet 15:

> באבונג ובלעז קמומילא וב״ח קבלי: חם דק והמבשלו במים ויכוף ראשו על אדו יתיך לחות המוח.

24 Cf. NM 2:12.

25 However, we disregarded the vocalization of the terminology in this Ms since it is, in our opinion, a later addition.

26 Cf. Johannes Uri, *Bibliothecae Bodleianae codicum manuscriptorum orientalium videlicet Hebraicorum, Chaldaicorum, Syriacorum, Aethiopicorum, Arabicorum, Persicorum, Turcicorum, Copticorumque Catalogus*, vol. 1 (Oxford: Clarendon, 1787), p. 106; Emilie Savage-Smith, *A New Catalogue of Arabic Manuscripts in the Bodleian Library, University of Oxford*, vol. 1, *Medicine* (Oxford: Oxford University Press, 2011), entry "42c," pp. 159–160. In our edition this Ms is indicated by the siglum O.

27 Such equivalences in other languages are called "synonyms" by the medieval authors themselves (cf. Guido Mensching and Gerrit Bos, "Arabic-Romance medico-botanical synonym lists in Hebrew manuscripts from the Iberian Peninsula and Italy (Vatican Library, fourteenth–fifteenth century)," in: *Aleph 15.1* (2015): 9–61, especially fn. no. 2, p. 9).

> *Bābūnağ* [i.e., Arab. for "chamomile" (*Matricaria chamomilla*)]; Rom. QMWMYL'; Rabb. Hebr. QBLY: It is hot [and] fine; if someone boils it in water and then bends his head over its vapor it will dissolve the humors in his brain.

The Romance/Latin terms are preceded by the Hebrew formula בלעז (*be-laʿaz*, 'in vernacular') or, in rare cases, by לטי' ('Latin'); they appear in approximately 85% of the entries, starting from Bet 6 onwards.[28] The fact that vernacular lexemes, written in Hebrew characters, are inserted in Hebrew texts, glossaries, and so-called synonym lists is a well-known phenomenon.[29] Shem Tov, born in Catalonia and active in southern France (cf. *supra*), had the intention to make the Jews, who did not master the Arabic language any longer, familiar with Arabic medicine and its terminology. In addition to the background described before in Chapter 1, it is worth mentioning that the ignorance of Arabic and the lack of a proper Hebrew terminology could lead the physicians to confuse ingredients of medical recipes.[30] To provide other physicians with the names of medicinal drugs and herbs in different languages, including Latin and vernacular languages, can thus be seen as a pragmatic and preventive measure on behalf of Shem Tov.[31] Although the Jews frowned upon Latin as the language of the Christian church, they often did not neatly distinguish between the vernacular Romance languages and Latin. As a consequence, Latin words are sometimes classifed as לעז and Romance words are sometimes labeled as לטי'. For the same reason, hybrid Latin–vernacular

28 The reason why they are absent before is not clear.

29 Cf., among others, Mensching and Savelsberg, *Manual*; Guido Mensching, "Eléments lexicaux et textes occitans en caractères hébreux," in: David Trotter (ed.), *Manuel de la philologie de l'édition* [= *Manuals of Romance Linguistics*, vol. 4], (Berlin, De Gruyter, 2015), pp. 237–264; Guido Mensching and Julia Zwink, "L'ancien occitan en tant que langage scientifique de la médecine. Termes vernaculaires dans la traduction hébraique du *Zad al-musafir wa-qut al-hadir* (XIIIe)," in: Carmen Alén Garbato et al. (ed.): *Los que fan viure e tresluire l'occitan. Actes du Xe congrès de l'AIEO, Béziers, 12–19 juin 2011*, pp. 226–236; Gerrit Bos and Guido Mensching, "A 15th Century Medico-Botanical Synonym List (Ibero-Romance-Arabic) in Hebrew Characters," in: *Panace@ 7.24* (2006); Mensching and Bos, "Arabic-Romance medico-botanical synonym lists."

30 Cf. Bos, Hussein, Mensching, and Savelsberg (eds.), *Medical Synonym Lists, Part 1*, p. 15.

31 Cf. Shem Tov's commentary to the second list of the *Sefer ha-Shimmush* (Bos, Kley, Mensching, and Savelsberg (eds.), *Medical Synonym Lists from Medieval Provence, Part 2*): "I have also composed an explanation of the drugs and herbs in vernacular and Arabic so that someone who goes on a distant journey will know their names in both languages."

terms appear now and then.[32] We will show some examples below, after having had a closer look at the linguistic nature of the terms labeled as *laʿaz* or Latin by Shem Tov.

Since Shem Tov lived in the Provence and translated the text for his Jewish compatriots of that region, it seems reasonable to assume that he uses the term *laʿaz* to designate Old Occitan, or more precisely, the Provençal dialect of this language. In fact, this has been shown to be the case for most of the vernacular items in the two synonym lists that appear as part of Shem Tov's *Sefer ha Shimmush*.[33] Occitan is a western Romance language that became famous through the poetry of the *trobadors*, who used a koiné commonly dubbed Old Provençal. Occitan subsists until today as a minority language in Southern France and small parts of Northern Spain and Northern Italy. Unsurprisingly, the vernacular that Shem Tov ben Isaac uses in the list edited in the present article also corresponds to Old Occitan, with some minor exceptions (words that are Catalan or French). For details, see the preliminary note to the supplement, which contains a detailed study of the Romance and Latin words that appear in the list.

The phenomenon of Old Occitan words, embedded in medical Hebrew texts and written in Hebrew characters, is not an isolated case. Many so-called synonym lists—precursors of bi- or multilingual medical lexicons—contain Old Occitan words, either because they were produced in Southern France or were based on Southern-French models.[34] As far as we know, Gerrit Bos and Guido Mensching, with their respective research groups, were the first to identify the language of most of the synonym lists as Old Occitan.[35] Before, the vernacular

---

32 Cf. Cyril Aslanov, "From Latin into Hebrew trough the Romance Vernaculars: the Creation of an Interlanguage Written in Hebrew Characters," in: Resianne Fontaine and Gad Freudenthal (ed.), *Latin-into-Hebrew: Texts and Studies*, vol. 1. (Leiden / Boston, Brill, 2013), pp. 69–84.

33 Cf. Bos, Hussein, Mensching, and Savelsberg (eds.), *Medical Synonym Lists, Part* 1, pp. 41–44.

34 Cf. Bos and Mensching, "Arabic-Romance medico-botanical synonym lists"; Gerrit Bos and Guido Mensching, "A Medico-Botanical Glossary in Hebrew Characters of Italian Origin (15th c., Ms. Florence, Med. Laur., Or. 17)," in: *Iberia Judaica VI* (2014), pp. 11–22; Dorothea Köhler and Guido Mensching, "Romanische Fachterminologie in mittelalterlichen medizinisch-botanischen Glossaren und Synonymenlisten in hebräischer Schrift," in: Laura Sergo et al. (edd.), *Fachsprache(n) in der Romania. Entwicklung, Verwendung, Übersetzung. XXXIIth Romanistentag, Berlin, September 2011* (Berlin, Frank & Timme, 2013), pp. 61–82.

35 Cf. Gerrit Bos and Guido Mensching, "Shem Tov Ben Isaac, Glossary of Botanical Terms, Nos. 1–18," in: *Jewish Quarterly Review* 92 (2001), pp. 21–40; Guido Mensching and Frank

words had often been uncritically identified as French or Spanish.[36] Another example is the case of entirely Hebrew texts, mostly translations from Arabic, containing Romance (mostly also Old Occitan) words that are often not identified as such and intergrated in the Hebrew text as a kind of technical loan words.[37]

In roughly 25% of the cases, the terms are not Romance but Latin. They are transcribed in the conventional way we know from other Latin texts or elements in Hebrew chracters.[38] In some cases, we find Romance–Latin hybrid terms (cf. above); see, e.g., בול שגלאטום (BWL ŠGL'ṬWM, Ṭet 2) for "sealed clay," composed of Romance *bol* and Lat. *sigillatum* or לנגא אויש (LNG' 'WYŠ, Lamed 7) for "ash tree," which is Romance *lenga* plus Latin *avis*.

With regard to their spelling and their meaning—i.e., their semantic equivalence to the Arabic and Hebrew terms—the vernacular terms are very often the same as those that we know from our studies on other medieval medical texts and synonym lists written in Hebrew characters. The resemblance of the vernacular lexemes of the *Sefer Almansur* to those of the two synonym lists of the *Sefer ha-Shimmush* is particularly conspicuous.[39] This is not surprising, since both works were written by the same author. Roughly speaking, 70% of

Savelsberg, "Reconstrucció de la terminologia mèdica occitanocatalana dels segles XIII i XIV a través de llistats de sinònims en lletres hebrees," in: Actes del congrès per a l'estudi dels Jueus en territori de llengua catalana, Barcelona-Girona 2001, ed. Josep Ribera-Florit, Barcelona: Universitat de Barcelona, Publicacions i Edicions, 2004, pp. 69–81; Gerrit Bos and Guido Mensching, "The Literature of Hebrew Medical Synonyms: Romance and Latin Terms and their Identification," in: *Aleph*: Historical Studies in Science and Judaism 5, 2005, pp. 169–211.

36 Cf. Bos, Hussein, Mensching, and Savelsberg (eds.), *Medical Synonym Lists, Part 1*; Bos and Mensching, "Shem Tov Ben Isaac, Glossary of Botanical Terms, Nos. 1–18."

37 Cf. Gerrit Bos, Guido Mensching, and Julia Zwink, *Romance Terms in Moses ibn Tibbon's* Ṣedat ha-derakhim, *the Hebrew Translation of Ibn al-Jazzār's* Zād al-musāfir wa-qūt al-ḥāḍir (*Book 7, Chap. 7–30*), (forthcoming); Guido Mensching and Julia Zwink, "L'ancien occitan en tant que langage scientifique." An example of a Latin-based Hebrew text that contains Romance words is the Hebrew version of *Macer Floridus*, see Gerrit Bos and Guido Mensching, "Macer Floridus: A Middle Hebrew Fragment with Romance Elements," in: *The Jewish Quarterly Review 16.1–2* (2000), pp. 17–51.

38 For the transcription of Latin words in Hebrew characters, cf. Bos, Hussein, Mensching, and Savelsberg (eds.), *Medical Synonym Lists, Part 1*, p. 44ff.; Cyril Aslanov, *Le provençal des Juifs et l'hébreu en Provence: le dictionnaire Šaršot ha-Kesef de Joseph Caspi*, Leuven-Paris, Peeters (2001); Lola Ferre, "La terminologia médica en las versiones hebreas de textos latinos," in: *Miscelánea de estudios árabes y hebraicos 40* (1991), pp. 87–107.

39 Bos, Hussein, Mensching, and Savelsberg (eds.), *Medical Synonym Lists, Part 1*; Bos, Kley, Mensching, and Savelsberg (eds.), *Medical Synonym Lists, Part 2*.

the vernacular terms that appear in the synonym list of the *Sefer Almansur* can also be found in at least one of the two synonym lists of the *Sefer ha-Shimmush*, and somewhat less in Ibn Tibbon's *Ṣedat ha-derakhim* (for details, see the supplement).

Hebrew Text and English Translation

אות האלף

1 אסרון: חם יבש מועיל מסתומי הכבד טוב לשקוי הבשר ומגיר השתן.

2 אפיתמון: חם ישלשל המרה השחורה ויסיר הנפח.

3 אדכר: חם יבש טוב למורסא הגסה באצטומכא והכבד כשיחובש בו.

4 אמיר באריס: קר מאמץ המעים מפסיק הצמא טוב לאצטומ׳ ושרשי השער.

5 אשק: חם יתיך המורסות הגסות כשיותך בחומץ ויחובש בו ויתיך החזירים.

6 אמלג׳: קר יבש מחזיק לאצטומכה ויכבה חומה וינגב הלחויות ויאות אל הטבע כלו והכבוש ממנו ירפה המעים ויועיל מרוחות השחורים ולבעל המרה השחורה ומן הליחה הלבנה ויוסיף בשכבת הזרע ויתן תאות המאכל ויפסיק הצמא.

7 אנגרא: חם יעורר תאות המשגל ויוציא הכיח מן החזה וישלשל הלחה הלבנה.

8 אשקיל: חם חד חריף מועיל מן הכפיון וגודל הטחול ולחישת האפעה והרנפלי הישן.

9 אפסנתין: חם יבש יחזק האצטומכה ויפתח סתומי הכבד ויועיל מן הקדחות הארוכות.

---

1 יבש: ב .om   4 ושרשי השער: والكبد الملتهبين O   6 אמלג׳: אלמוג א || ויכבה ... הצמא: وأصول الشعر O   7 אנגרא: אלנגרא א   8 חד: جدا O   9 ויפתח: ויחזק א

Alef

1 Asarabacca (*Asarum Europaeum*): It is hot [and] dry; it is beneficial for obstructions of the liver, good for dropsy of the flesh, and makes the urine flow.

2 Dodder (*Cuscuta epithymum Murray* and Var.): It is hot, purges black bile, and dispels tumors.

3 Camel grass (*Cymbopogon schoenanthus*): It is hot [and] dry, good for a hard tumor in the stomach and liver when it is applied as a poultice to it.

4 Barberry (*Berberis vulgaris*): It is cold, it constipates the bowels, lessens thirst, [and] is good for the stomach and the roots of the hair.

5 Gum ammoniac (a product of *Dorema Ammoniacum Don.*): It is hot; it dissolves hard tumors when it is dissolved in vinegar and applied as a poultice to them; it also dissolves scrofula.

6 Emblic myrobalan (fruit of *Phyllanthus Emblica*): It is cold [and] dry, it strengthens the stomach and cools its heat; it dries the humors and is good for one's whole nature (constitution); [when taken as] a conserve it loosens the bowels and is beneficial for winds [caused by] black bile, and for a melancholic person, and phlegm; it increases the sperm and appetite and lessens thirst.

7 Roman nettle (*Urtica pilulifera*): It is hot, awakens sexual lust, expels sputum from the chest and purges phlegm.

8 Sea squill (*Drimia maritima*, synonym: *Scilla maritima*): It is very hot [and] sharp, it is beneficial for epilepsy, for an enlarged spleen, for viper bites, and for chronic asthma.

9 Absinth/wormwood (*Artemisia absinthium*): It is hot [and] dry, strengthens the stomach and opens obstructions of the liver, and is beneficial for chronic fevers.

---

1 "Asarabacca" (ʾSRWN): Cf. IĞ 9. 2 "Dodder" (ʾPYTMWN): Cf. IĞ 807. 3 "Camel grass" (ʾDKR): Cf. IĞ 181. 4 "Barberry" (ʾMYR BʾRYS): Cf. IĞ 86. || "stomach and the roots of the hair": Cf. O: "inflamed stomach and liver"; "and the roots of the hair" features under entry "emblic myrobalan." 5 "Gum ammoniac" (ʾŠQ): Cf. IĞ 3. 6 "Emblic myrobalan" (ʾMLĞ): Cf. IĞ 951. || "It … thirst": Cf. O: "it strengthens the stomach and the roots of the hair." 7 "Roman nettle" (ʾNGRʾ): Cf. IĞ 16. 8 "Sea squill" (ʾŠQYL): Cf. IĞ 35. || "viper bites": Lit., "the hissing of vipers." || "asthma" (רנפלי): Cf. NM 2:19. 9 "Absinth/wormwood" (ʾPSNTYN): Cf. IĞ 452.

10 אסטוכודוס: חם ישלשל המרה השחורה והליחה הלבנה ויועיל מן הכפיון והשגעון כשירבו השלשול בו.

11 אכליל אלמלך: חם מרכך המורסות הגסות בפרקים ובכסלים.

12 אניסון: חם יגרש הרוחות ויפתח סתומי הכבד ויסכסך תאות המשגל.

13 אקאקיא: קר יבש מפסיק הדם ישיב בליטת פי הטבעת ויאמץ המעים.

14 אפיון: קר יבש מקדיר מישן ומשקיט מסלת(?) האברים המחוממים ומונע התחדש המורסה.

15 אשנה: מעוטת החמימות תעצור הקיא ותחזק האצטומכה.

16 אתמד: קר יבש מחזק העין שומר בריאותה ויועיל עוד מהגרת דם הנדות כשתשא ממנו האשה.

17 אנזרות: טוב לצואת העין והאפר והחבורות הטריות.

18 אנפחה: כלן חמות מאמצות המעים אומץ חזק ומפסיקות רעיפת הדם.

19 אבהל: חם יבש מגיר השתן בחזקה ומפיל העובר.

20 אספידאג: קר יבש קובץ ומנגב הלחות ומצמיח הבשר.

21 אירסא והיא שרשי השושן יועיל מעקיצת הרמשים וינקה החזה והריאה.

---

10 אסטוכודוס: אסטלפירוס א ‖ והשגעון: والمالنخوليا O 11 ובכסלים: والأحشاء O 12 ויסכסך: ويحرّك O 14 אפיון ... המורסה: om. O ‖ מסלת(?): ומלחלחי(?) ב ‖ המורסה: om. א 15 מעוטת: מעוט ב 16 ויועיל: ويقطع ويسقط O ‖ כשתשא: اذا احتمل O 17 לצואת: للرمص O ‖ והאפר: والرمد O 18 מאמצות המעים: تعقل البطن O 19 השתן: الطمث O 20 אספידאג: אספירא א אספידאג ... הבשר: om. O 21 אירסא ... והריאה: om. O

10 French lavender (*Lavendula stoechas*): It is hot, purges black bile and phlegm, and is beneficial for epilepsy and melancholy when it is applied frequently as a purgative.

11 Melilot/king's clover (*Melilotus officinalis*): It is hot; it softens hard tumors in the joints and loins.

12 Anise (*Pimpinella anisum*): It is hot; it dispels winds, opens obstructions of the liver, and stimulates the libido.

13 Acacia gum (Senegal gum): It is cold and dry; it stops bleeding, reduces a protruding anus, and constipates the bowels.

14 Opium: It is cold [and] dry; it is a narcotic and soporific, calms (soothes) [...] feverish limbs, and prevents the occurrence of tumors (inflammations).

15 Lichen (*Alectoria usneoides*): It has little [warming properties]; it checks vomiting and strengthens the stomach.

16 Stibium: It is cold [and] dry; it strengthens the eye [and] preserves its health; it is also beneficial for menstrual bleeding when the woman applies it as a suppository.

17 Sarcocol (gum resin of *Astragalus sarcocolla*): It is beneficial for rheum in the eye, ophthalmia, and fresh wounds.

18 Rennet: All [sorts of rennet] are hot; they constipate the bowels in a severe way and stop a nosebleed.

19 Savin juniper (*Juniperus sabina*): It is hot [and] dry; it makes the urine flow with force and causes a miscarriage.

20 White lead: It is cold, dry, astringent; it dries the humors and closes [wounds] up.

21 Iris (the white Florentine iris [*Iris germanica var. florentina*] and the Spanish iris [*Iris xiphium*]); i.e., the rhizome of the iris: It is beneficial for stings and bites of vermin and it cleanses the chest and lungs.

---

10 "French lavender" (ʾSṬWKWDWS): Cf. IĞ 28. ‖ "melancholy" (שגעון): As a rule, Shem Tov translates Arabic مالنخوليا as Hebrew שטות (cf. SHS 1:514 [Shin 31]; NM 2:117) or שגעון, which have the standard meaning of "madness, folly." 11 "Melilot/king's clover" (ʾKLYL ʾLMLK): Cf. IĞ 50. 12 "Anise" (ʾNYSWN): Cf. IĞ 384. ‖ "stimulates" (יסכסך): Cf. NM 2:16. 13 "Acacia gum" (ʾQʾQYʾ): Cf. IĞ 51. 14 "Opium ... tumors (inflammations)": Missing in O. 15 "Lichen" (ʾŠNH): Cf. IĞ 49. 16 "Stibium" (ʾTMD): Cf. KM 1:205–210. ‖ "is also beneficial for": Cf. O: "also stops." 17 "Sarcocol" (ʾNZRWT): Cf. IĞ 477. ‖ "rheum" (צואת העין): Cf. NM 2:17. ‖ "ophthalmia" (אפר): Cf. NM 2:10. 18 "Rennet" (ʾNPḤH): Cf. IĞ 78. 19 "Savin juniper" (ʾBHL): Cf. IĞ 27. ‖ "the urine": Cf. O: "the menstrual blood." 20 "White lead" (ʾSPYDʾG): Cf. KM 1:241–246; "White ... up": Om. O. 21 "Iris" (ʾYRSʾ): Cf. IĞ 1. ‖ "iris" (ŠWŠN): Hebrew ŠWŠN normally means "lily," but in this context also "iris," after Arabic *sawsan*; cf. SHS 1:511–512 (Shin 27); for "rhizome of the iris," cf. IĞ 1: وقال أهرن الإ يرسا هو أصول السوسن الذي على لون السماء (Ahrun: *īrisā* is the rhizome of the sky-blue iris).

22 אלבאלילג: יבש אוכל הבשר והמרה ומעבד האסטומכה.

אות הבית

1 בלסאן: חם שמנו ועצו יועילו מלחישת האפעה והעקרב ומכאב הרחם.

2 בנג: מחמם ומקדיר והשחור יותר חזק ואפשר שימית והדך אותו ומחבש בו המורסות החזקות הדפיקה מקדיר אותם ומשקיטם.

3 ברשיאושן: חם והשורף אותו ונותן דשנו על שער הראש וילפף ומלפלף אותו יצמיח השער ויתיך החזירים וינקה הריאה מן החלטים העבים המסתבכים בה.

4 בהמן: יש ממנו אדום ויש ממנו לבן חמים מעוררים תאות המשגל.

5 בוזידאן: חם יוסיף בתאוה וימנע מן הפודגרא.

6 בסבאיג ובלעז פוליפודיאו: חם משלשל המרה השחורה ומתיך ההדרוקן כשילקח עם המרק.

7 בלבוס הוא בצל נאכל: יסכסך תאות המשגל וכשיוטח בו הפנים יסיר בו הנתק.

---

22 אלבאלילג: emend. ed. אלבאליג א אלבאכליג ב אלבאלילג ... האסטומכה: om. O

1 חם: حبّه O 2 בנג: בנו א ‖ מחמם ומקדיר: מקמר וגורם תונבא א جميع أصنافه مسكّرة مخدّرة O ‖ והדך אותו: وإذا دقّ O ‖ החזקות: emend. ed. מ(?) חזק א ⟨...⟩ ב ‖ מקדיר אותם ומשקיטם: أبطل حسّها O 3 וילפף: emend. ed. ומלפלף א ⟨...⟩ ב وتغلف O 5 בתאוה: في الباه O 6 ההדרוקן: القولنج O ‖ כשילקח עם המרק: om. O 7 בלבוס ... הנתק: om. O

22 Beleric myrobalan (*Terminalia bellirica*): It is dry; it corrodes the flesh and the bile and strengthens the stomach.

Bet

1 Balsam tree (*Commiphora opobalsamum*): It is hot; its oil and wood are beneficial for bites of vipers and stings of scorpions and for pain in the womb.

2 Black henbane (*Hyoscyamus niger var. albus*): It has a heating and narcotic effect; the black [variety] is stronger and possibly fatal; if it is pounded and applied as a poultice on abscesses that are severely pulsating it benumbs and abates them.

3 Maidenhair fern (*Adiantum capillus Veneris*): It is hot; it makes the hair of the head grow if one burns it and puts its ashes on [the hair] and covers [the hair] with it; it dissolves scrofula and cleanses the lungs from thick humors that got stuck in them.

4 Behen: There is a red [variety] (identified by some modern authors as *Statice limonium*) and a white [variety] (*Centaurea behen*); they are hot and arouse the sexual lust.

5 BWZYD'N (*būzīdān*): It is hot, it strengthens the libido and prevents [the occurrence] of podagra.

6 Common polypody (*Polypodium vulgare*); Romance PWLYPWDY'W: It is hot, it purges black bile and cures a colic when it is taken [in a decoction].

7 BLBWS; i.e., an edible onion (tassel hyacinth, *Leopoldia comosa*, synonym: *Muscari comosum*): It stimulates the sexual lust and when it is smeared on the face it removes the freckles.

---

22 "Beleric myrobalan" ('LB'LYLG): Cf. IĞ 1028. || "strengthens" (מעבד): Cf. NM 2:16.

1 "Balsam tree" (BLS'N): Cf. IĞ 155. || "it is hot, its oil and wood": Cf. O: "Its fruit, wood and oil." 2 "Black henbane" (BNG): Cf. IĞ 655. || "It has a heating and narcotic effect": Cf. O: "All of its species have an intoxicating and narcotic effect." || "narcotic effect" (מקדיר): Cf. NM 2:17–18. 3 "Maidenhair fern" (BRŠY'WŠN): Cf. IĞ 133. 4 "Behen" (BHMN): Cf. DT 4:91 (n. 9). 5 "BWZYD'N (*būzīdān*)": Although identified by most Arabic and Persian physicians with *ḫuṣā aṯ-ṯaʿlab* (lit., "fox testicles," a common name of orchids), its true identity is hard to establish; cf. DT 4:8, n. 5; M 56; IĞ 292. 6 "Common polypody" (BSB'YG): Cf. IĞ 119; SHS 1:368–369 (Samekh 32). || "colic": Arab. قولنج is translated by Shem Tov with Hebrew הדרוקן, which is the regular term for "dropsy"; cf. NM 2:11. || "when it is taken [in a decoction]": Om. O. 7 "BLBWS": Cf. IĞ 115. || "BLBWS … freckles": Om. O. || "stimulates" (יסכסך): Cf. Alef 12 above.

8 באדאורדי ובלעז קורויולא או קורגיולא וב״ח קיסוס: יועיל ויבריא מן הקדחות הישנות.

9 ברנגמשך הוא אלחבק אלקרנפל ובלע׳ אוזימו גירופלא: חם יבש יועיל מעובי הטחול ויסיר הקושי.

10 באן ובלעז ישמין: ירכך המורסא הגסה ויתיכה ויסיר הנתק כשיוטח בו הפנים ושמנו טוב לעובי הנשאר מרושם החיבוש וירכך המורסות היבשות ויחמם העצבים רע לאצטומכה גורם אסטניסות ורפיון מעים.

11 בסד: קר יבש מועיל כשישחק היטב וישתה מרקיקת הדם ומחזק העין ומפסיק הדמעה.

12 בלאדור: חם יבש מאד יועיל מן החליים הקרים ⟨ו⟩השכחה אלא שהוא ישרוף הדם ואפשר שיעורר שטות.

13 בזרקטונא ובלעז שליום וכשישתה באישרוב גלאבי תכבה החום ותשקיט הלהבה ותרכך החזה ותועיל מן העיצום אשר יהיה במעים והטורף אותה בחומץ ויחובש בה המפצלים כשיהיה בהם מורסות חמות תשקיט אותם ר״ל תשקיט כאבם.

---

8 יועיל: في الحرارة ما هو نافع O 9 ברנגמשך ... הקושי: om. O 10 נתק: كلف O ‖ מרושם: מעובי א ‖ המורסות: الأوتار O ‖ גורם אסטניסות ורפיון מעים: مطلق للبطن O 11 בסד ... הדמעה: om. O 12 בלאדור: בורק ובלעז שלניטרי א ‖ שטות: وسواس O 13 באישרוב: באשירוב א באישרוב גלאבי: بجلاب O ‖ ותועיל מן העיצום אשר יהיה במעים: om. א ‖ במעים: اذا قلي وشرب add. O ‖ המפצלים: המפלצים א

8 Scotch thistle (*Onopordum acanthium*, or perhaps soldier thistle [*Picnomon acarna*]), Rom. QWRWYWL' or QWRGYWL', and Rabb. Hebr. QYSWS (ivy, *Hedera helix*): It is beneficial for chronic fevers and it cures them.

9 BRNGMŠK (*barangǧamušk*) (a type of basil or mint, that cannot be identified); i.e., *al-ḥabaq al-qaranfulī*; Rom. 'WZYMW GYRWPL': It is hot [and] dry; it is beneficial for thickness of the spleen (enlarged spleen) and removes its hardness.

10 Ben [-oil tree] (*Moringa oleifera Lam*); Rom. YŠMYN: It softens and dissolves a hard tumor and removes freckles when it is rubbed on the face; its oil is good for the thickness that remains from the setting [of a fracture?]. It softens dry tendons and heats the nerves, [but] it is bad for the stomach as it causes nausea and looseness of the bowels.

11 Coral: It is hot [and] dry; when it is well pounded and then ingested it is beneficial for hemoptysis; it strengthens the eye and stops a continuous weeping discharge (rhyas).

12 Marking nut (*Semecarpus anacardium*): It is very hot [and] dry; it is beneficial for cold diseases and for forgetfulness; however, it burns the blood and sometimes causes delusion (delirium).

13 Fleawort/psyllium seed (*Plantago afra*, synonym: *Plantago psyllium*); Rom. ŠLYWM: It brings down the fever and its burning heat when it is ingested with juleb syrup, and it softens the chest. It is good for intestinal illness (dysentery) [when it is roasted and ingested]. If it is mixed with vinegar and applied as a poultice to the joints—when these are afflicted by inflamed tumors—it abates them, i.e., it alleviates their pain.

---

8 "Scotch thistle" (B'D'WRDY): Cf. IǦ 133. ‖ "Rom. QWRWYWL' … QYSWS": Cf. SHS 1:461 (Qof 23). 9 "BRNGMŠK (*barangǧamušk*)": Cf. IǦ 64, 154; "BRNGMŠK … hardness": Om. O. ‖ "*al-ḥabaq al-qaranfulī*": Was often considered to be a synonym for *barangǧamušk*; cf. DT 3:43; IǦ 154. 10 "Ben oil tree" (B'N): Cf. IǦ 970. ‖ "freckles" (נתק; Arab. كلف): Cf. NM 2:15–16. ‖ "setting [of a fracture]" (חיבוש): Cf. NM 2:12. ‖ "tendons": Translated after O; Shem Tov: "tumors." ‖ "it causes nausea and looseness of the bowels": "it relieves the bowels" O. ‖ "nausea" (אסטניסות): Cf. NM 2:30. 11 "Coral" (BSD): Cf. IǦ 111; "Coral … (rhyas)": Om. O. ‖ "a continuous weeping discharge (rhyas)" (דמעה): Cf. NM 2:11. 12 "Marking nut" (BL'DWR): Cf. IǦ 2; see also Gerrit Bos, "Baladhur (Marking-nut): A popular medieval drug for strengthening memory," *Bulletin of the School of Oriental and African Studies*, 59, no. 2 (1996): 229–236. ‖ "delusion (delirium)" (שטות): Cf. NM 2:19. For its use in the sense of "melancholy," see Alef 10 above. 13 "Fleawort/psyllium" (BZRQṬWN'): Cf. IǦ 8; IT, Shin 1. ‖ "intestinal illness (dysentery)" (העיצום אשר יהיה במעים): Cf. NM 2:16. ‖ "[when it is roasted and ingested]": Translated after O. ‖ "joints" (מפצלים): Cf. NM 2:14.

14 בנגנכסת ובלעז אנוש קאשטוש וקוראים אותו ישמעאל אילן אברהם: חם יבש מועיל מעובי הטחול ויסיר הקושי.

15 באבונג ובלעז קמומילא ובי"ח קבלי: חם דק והמבשלו במים ויכוף ראשו על אדו יתיך לחות המות.

אות הגימל

1 גוז מאתל בומיטא: חם טוב מעקיצת עקרב וגורם שכרות וקיא ואפשר שימית.

2 גאושיר ובלעז אפופונק: חם מאד מגרש הרוחות טוב למי שתקרנה לו רוחות עבות ומועיל למכאובי הרחמים.

3 געדה ובלעז פוליום מונטנום ובי"ח סיאה: חמה גורמת מיחוש בראש טוב לקדחות הישנות הקרות ואל השקוי והירקון ותועיל מעקיצת העקרבים.

4 גנטיאנה ובלעז גנסיאנה: חמה יבשה מאמצה המעים טובה לעקיצת העקרב והכבד הקר והסתום והטחול העב.

5 גבסין ובלעז גיף החרסית קר יבש יפסיק הדם כשטורפין אותו בחלמון ביצה ויושת על החבורה ואם ישתה ימית.

---

14 בנגנכסת: בנגנסת ב ‖ מעובי: om. O 15 באבונג ... המוח: om. O

1 בומיטא: emend. ed. נומיטא א ‖ חם טוב מעקיצת עקרב: مخدّر O 2 הרחמים: الأرحام الباردة O
3 געדה: גוערה א ‖ מונטנום: מונטדום א ‖ חמה: om. א ‖ טוב: om. א ‖ הקרות: om. O 4 גנטיאנה ... העב: om. ב ‖ גנסיאנה: emend. ed. גיסיאנה א ‖ מאמצה המעים: om. O 5 גבסין: גלרסין א

14 Chaste tree (*Vitex agnus castus*); Rom. ʾNWŠ Qʾ ŠṬWŠ, and the Arabs call it "tree of Abraham": It is hot [and] dry; it is beneficial for thickness of the spleen (enlarged spleen) and stops an erection.

15 Chamomile (*Matricaria chamomilla*); Rom. QMWMYLʾ; Rabb. Hebr. QBLY: It is hot [and] fine; if someone boils it in water and then bends his head over its vapor it will dissolve the humors in his brain.

Gimel

1 Metel nut (*Datura metel*); [Rom.] BWMYṬʾ: It is hot [and] good for scorpion stings; it causes intoxication and vomiting and can be fatal.

2 Opopanax (i.e., the concreted resin of *Opopanax chironium Koch*); Rom. ʾPWPWNQ: It is very hot; it expels winds; it is good for someone affected by thick winds, and it is beneficial for pains in the womb.

3 Germander (*Teucrium sp*, especially the felty germander [*Teucrium polium*]); Rom. PWLYWM MWNṬNWM; Rabb. Hebr. SYʾH: It is hot [and] causes headache; it is good for chronic fevers, dropsy, jaundice, and beneficial for scorpion stings.

4 Gentian (*Gentiana lutea*); Rom. GNSYʾNH: It is hot [and] dry; it constipates the bowels; it is good for scorpion stings, for a cold and blocked liver, and thick spleen.

5 Gypsum; Rom. GYP (of clay): It is cold [and] dry; it stops the bleeding [of a wound] when it is mixed with egg yolk and put on [it]; it is fatal when one ingests it.

---

14 "Chaste tree" (BNGNKST): Cf. SHS 1:114–115 (Alef 30). ‖ "erection" (קושי): Cf. Arabic إنعاظ.
15 "Chamomile" (Bʾ BWNG): Cf. IĞ 24; SHS 1:456–457 (Qof 15); "Chamomile … brain": Om. O.

1 "Metel nut (*Datura metel*), [Rom.] BWMYṬʾ": Cf. SHS 1:102 (Alef 15); IĞ 199. ‖ "It is hot [and good] for scorpion stings": Cf. O: "It has a narcotic effect." 2 "Opopanax" (Gʾ WŠYR): Cf. IĞ 81; IT, Alef 23. ‖ "womb": Cf. O: "cold womb." 3 "Germander" (GʿDH): Cf. IĞ 193; SHS 1:363–364 (Samekh 20). ‖ "chronic fevers": Translated acc. to O (cf. IB 1: 224; IBF 1: no. 488: "Razès. Elle est salutaire contre les fièvres chroniques et les piqûres de scorpions"); Shem Tov has: "chronic cold fevers." 4 "Gentian" (GNṬYʾNH): Cf. IĞ 214; IT, Gimel 8; "Gentian … spleen": Om. ב. ‖ "it constipates the bowels": Om. O. 5 "Gypsum" (GBSYN): Cf. KM 1:247–249; SHS 1:152 (Gimel 10).

6 גלבהנק: חם מקיא בכח חזק ויועיל לבעלי הפלג כשיקיאו בו ופעולתו קרובה מפעולת האליברוס והלקיחה ממנו משקל דרכמון ואפשר שימית בכח הקיא.

7 גלנאר לע׳ בלאושטיאש: קר יבש מאמץ המעים ועוצר הדם.

8 גודואר אלזנכבאר ובלע׳ סיטול: כחו כח הזרנבאד: יש בו מותר חם יועיל מן הרוחות ⟨ו⟩מעקיצת הרמשים אלא שהוא יותר דק מן הזרנבאד.

9 גנדבא דסתר ובלעז קשטור: חם מחמם העצבים ומגיר דם הנדות ומתיך הנפח וההדרוקן.

10 גוזבוא הוא אגוז מושקדא: חם טוב לכבד והאצטומכה הקרים מאמץ המעים.

11 גאריקון ובלעז אגריק: חם פותח האטמים מן הכבד הקר ומועיל מן הכפיון ומשלשל החלטים העבים והוא טוב לטבע.

12 גאפת בלעז נאשקא או ח(א)ריבברא: חם פותח סיתומי הכבד טוב מן הקדחות הישנות.

---

6 גלבהנק: גלבהק א جبلهنك O ‖ קרובה מפעולת: ב .om ‖ והלקיחה: وأكثر ما يسقا O 7 בלאושטיאש: קפיל דגלנש א ‖ קר יבש: א .om ‖ מאמץ המעים ועוצר הדם: יועיל מרפיון האצטומכה והרחם כשיבושל וישבו בו א ‖ הדם: ורבויו ימית ב .add 8 גודואר ... יותר דק מן הזרנבאד: O .om ‖ כחו כח הזרנבאד: יש בו מותר חם יועיל מן הרוחות ⟨ו⟩מעקיצת הרמשים אלא שהוא יותר דק מן הזרנבאד: א .om ‖ הזרנבאד: .emend. ed הזרנבת ב 9 גנדבא דסתר ... וההדרוקן: O .om ‖ וההדרוקן: וההדרוקון ב 10 חם: يابس O .add ‖ טוב לכבד והאצטומכה הקרים מאמץ המעים: .emend. ed טוב לכבד מאמץ המעים והאצטומכה הקרים אב يعقل البطن جيّد للمعدة والكبد الباردتين O 11 הקר: O .om ‖ מן הכפיון: للربو والصرع O

6 Wild sesame (*Reseda alba*): It is hot; it induces violent vomiting; it is beneficial for hemiplegia patients when it makes them vomit; its effect is similar to that of hellebore (*Helleborus albus* or *Veratrum album* and *Helleborus niger*); the [maximum] dosis one may take is one *dirham*. It may kill through the violence of the vomiting.

7 Pomegranate flower (*Punica granatum*); Rom. BL'WŠṬY'Š: It is cold [and] dry; it constipates the bowels and stops bleeding.

8 Zedoary (*Curcuma zedoaria*) ZNKB'R; Rom. SYṬWL: Its power is [similar to] that of bitter ginger (shampoo ginger, *Zingiber zerumbet*): It has a hot [substance] that is beneficial for winds and for the stings and bites of vermin; however, it is more gentle than bitter ginger.

9 Castoreum; Rom. QŠṬWR: It is hot; it heats the nerves and induces menstruation and dissolves swellings and [cures] a colic.

10 Nutmeg (the seed of *Myristica fragrans Houtt.*); i.e., [Hebr. Rom.] 'GWZ MWŠQD': It is hot [and] good for a cold liver and stomach; it constipates the bowels.

11 Agaric (*Fomes officinalis*); Rom. 'GRYQ: It is hot; it opens obstructions in a cold liver, is beneficial for epilepsy, purges thick humors, and is good for one's nature (constitution).

12 Agrimony (*Agrimonia eupatoria*); Rom. N'SQ' or Ḥ('?)RYBBR': It is hot, it opens obstructions of the liver, [and] it is good for chronic fevers.

---

6 "Wild sesame" (GLBHNQ): Cf. IĞ 200. ‖ "hellebore": Cf. SHS 1:213 (Ḥet 8). ‖ "the [maximum] dosis": Cf. O. ‖ "*dirham*": The standard *dirham* is 3.125 grams; see Walther Hinz, *Islamische Masse und Gewichte, umgerechnet ins metrische System: Photomechanischer Nachdruck mit Zusätzen und Berichtigungen*, = *Handbuch der Orientalistik* 1, Ergänzungsband 1.1 (Leiden: Brill, 1970), p. 3. 7 "Pomegranate flower" (GLN'R): Cf. IĞ 212; IT, Bet 6. ‖ "it constipates the bowels and stops bleeding": Cf. א: "it is good for feebleness of the stomach and uterus when one boils it and sits in the [boiled extract]." ‖ "bleedings": ב adds, "but it is fatal in an overdose." 8 "Zedoary" (GWDW'R); Cf. IĞ 206: جدوار هو الزرنباد في قول بعض الناس، وقال عليّ بن رزين في كتاب الفردوس: هو مثل الزرنباد ⟨في القوة⟩ وألطف منه، وفي الحاوي: هو قطع تشبه الزرنباد. *Al-ǧadwār* (zedoary) is the bitter ginger (*zurunbād*), according to the assertion of some people. 'Alī ibn Razīn in his book entitled "The Paradise" (*Kitāb al-Firdaws*): It is similar to the *zurunbād*, ⟨as regards power⟩, but more gentle. (Sc. al-Rāzī's) *Ḥāwī*: It consists of pieces resembling the *zurunbād*. ‖ "ZNKB'R": Read: ZNĞB'R? ("Zanzibar"). 9 "Castoreum" (GNDB' DSTR): I.e., an excretion of the scent glands of the European beaver (*Castor fiber*); cf. IĞ 183; "Castoreum ... colic": Om. O. ‖ "colic" (HDRWQN): Cf. entry Bet 6 above. 10 "Nutmeg" (GWZBW'): Cf. IĞ 192. ‖ "hot": "[and] dry" add. O. ‖ "good for a cold liver and stomach; it constipates the bowels": emend. ed. (following O): "good for the liver; it constipates the cold bowels and stomach" אב. 11 "Agaric" (G'RYQWN): Cf. IT, Alef 2. ‖ "obstructions" (אטמים): Cf. NM 2:9. ‖ "cold": Om O. ‖ "for epilepsy": Cf. O: "for asthma and epilepsy." 12 "Agrimony" (G'PYT): Cf. IĞ 182.

13 גרא אלגלוד ובלע׳ גלות: טוב לשעפה והפיתקה ורקיקת הדם.

14 גרב ובלע׳ שלזין: כששורפין קליפתו ויתן דשנו על היבלות ינתקם.

15 גאר ובלעז לורוש: טוב למורסות הרחם ולעקיצת העקרבים ומכאובי העצבים גרגריו ושמנו.

אות הדלת

1 דרונג: חם טוב לרוחות העבות ולמכאובי הרחמים הקרים ודפיקת הלב מן הקרירות ועקיצת העקרבים.

2 דפלא ובלעז לורדמוני וב״ח הרדפוני: חמה טובה לגרב ולחכוך הורגת החמורים והבהמות ובני אדם אם יאכלו ממנו וטובה לכאב הברכים והגב הישנים כשיחובש בה.

3 דבק ובלע׳ וישק וב״ח דבק: חם מנגב המורסות.

4 דארשישעאן: חם קובץ טוב לשחין הפה למתגרגר במים שנתבשל בהם או לגמוע הפה בהם מועיל ⟨מקושי⟩ השתן והנפח ורפיון העצבים והמבשלו ביין וטובל בו פתילה ויכניסה באף יועיל מן הסרחון המתהוה בו.

---

13 אלגלוד: אלגילוד א الجلود O || לשעפה: للسعفة O והקיא א add. 14 כששורפין: כששותין א כששורפין ... ינתקם: نافع من استطلاق البطن والقلاع غاية النفع O 15 ושמנו: ويغثي ويقيّئ O add.

1 מן: מע O || ועקיצת: ולעקיצת ב 2 דפלא: דלפה א || והגב: והגרב ב 3 חם מנגב: حارّ يابس يفشّ O 4 לשחין הפה: للقلاع O || או לגמוע הפה בהם: ב om. O || מועיל: emend. ed. מערוב א מועיל ... ורפיון: ב om. || ורפיון: emend. ed. והכפיון אב

13 Glue from skins; Rom. GLWṬ: It is good for cradle cap, hernia, and hemoptysis.

14 Willow or poplar (esp. the species *Salix babylonica*, or *Populus Euphratica Oliv.*); Rom. ŠLZYN: It uproots warts if one burns its rind and puts the ashes on them.

15 Laurel (*Laurus nobilis*); Rom. LWRWŠ: Its berries and oil are good for tumors of the uterus, scorpion stings and painful nerves (neuralgia).

Dalet

1 Leopard's bane (*Doronicum pardalianches*): It is hot [and] good for thick winds, for cold uterine pains, for palpitations of the heart caused by cold, and for scorpion stings.

2 Oleander (*Nerium Oleander or. Var.*); Rom. LWRDMWNY; Rabb. Heb. HRDPWNY: It is hot [and] good for mange and for itch; it kills donkeys and [other] animals and human beings when they eat therefrom; when it is applied as a poultice it is good for chronic pain in the knees and back.

3 Bird-lime; Rom. WYŠQ; Rabb. Heb. DBQ: It is hot [and] dries tumors.

4 D'RŠYŠ''N: It is hot [and] astringent, [and] when one applies a decoction of it as a gargle, it is good for ulcers in the mouth; it is beneficial for dysuria, flatulence, and feebleness of the nerves; it is good for the stench developing inside the nose when it is dipped and boiled in wine and inserted in it as a suppository.

---

13 "Cradle cap": Arab. سعفة; cf. UW 156, s.v. ἀχώρ (cf. LS 298: "scurf, dandruff") and 344, s.v. κηρίον (LS 948: "honeycomb, II. a cutaneous disease μελικηρίς"; cf. LS 1097: "a kind of cyst or wen, from its resembling a honeycomb"): "böser Grind": for this affection see also Al-Rāzī, *On the Treatment of Small Children* (*De curis puerorum*)*: The Latin and Hebrew Translations*, eds. and trans. Gerrit Bos and Michael McVaugh (Leiden: Brill, 2015), p. 20, 31, 48, 66. ‖ "hernia" (PYTQH): Cf. NM 2:17. 14 "Willow" (GRB): Cf. IĞ 798; SHS 1:388–389 (Ayin 16). ‖ "It … them": Cf. O: "It is extremely beneficial for diarrhea and for aphthae." 15 "Laurel" (G'R): Cf. IĞ 1089; IT, Lamed 1. ‖ "painful nerves (neuralgia)": "and it causes nausea and vomiting" add. O.

1 "Leopard's bane" (DRWNG): Cf. DT 4:68, n. 14. ‖ "palpitations of the heart" (דפיקת הלב): The Hebrew term can also refer to "heartburn"; cf. NM 3:53. ‖ "caused": Cf. O: "accompanied." 2 "Oleander" (DPL'): Cf. IĞ 388; SHS 1:182–183 (He 3). ‖ "mange" (גרב): The Hebrew term can also refer to "trachoma" cf. NM 2:177. 3 "Bird-lime" (DBQ): Cf. D 1:424. 4 "D'RŠYŠ''N" (*dāršīšaʿān*): The plant called "aspalathos" by Dioscurides; it designates different species of Cytisus, Sarothamnus, Ulex, Genistella, Genista, and Spartium; cf. DT 1:17; M 88; IĞ 223. ‖ "ulcers in the mouth": Cf. O: "aphthae." ‖ "it is beneficial for dysuria, flatulence, and feebleness": Om. ב.

5 דלב ובלעז פושטא: עליו ואגוזיו קרים יבשים והשוחק אותם בחומץ ומחבש בו שרפת האש יועילהו והמבשל קלפתו בחומץ ומגמע בו הפה יועיל ממכאובי השינים.

6 דרדי אלכמר וב״מ שמרי היין: חם וישקיט המורסות החמות ויתיכם כשיוטח בו עליהם. ודורדיא של חומץ לא יחמם וישקיט המורסות החמות כשיוטח עליהם.

7 דכאן ר״ל קטרת: קטורת הדברים תשוב אל פעולת מה שיצמח ממנה ובכלל כי כל קטורת חמה יבשה ותכונתה מה שיתילד ממנה.

8 דם אלאכוין ובלעז שנג דראגין: קר מאמץ המעים ומדביק החבורות הלחות הטריות.

9 דראריח ובלעז קנטרידש וב״ח מאירות: חמים חדים טובים לגרב ואם ישתה מהם הרבה יעשו שחין בכיס מקוה המים וגורמים השתות דם ואפשר שימיתו והמעט מהם יגיר השתן.

10 דנב אלכיל זנב הסוס ובלעז קודא דקאבל: קר טוב לשלשול הבטן ורקיקת הדם והמורסות החמות.

11 דהב זהב ובלעז אור: טוב לדפיקת הלב והשתוממות הנפש.

---

5 ומגמע בו הפה: وتمضمض به O || ממכאובי: מכאב ב 6 אלכמר: אליכמר א || וישקיט המורסות החמות ויתיכם כשיוטח בו עליהם: محلّل الأورام O 7 דכאן ... מה שיתילד ממנה: om. O 8 אלאכוין: אלכוין א 9 דראריח ... השתן: om. O || השתות דם: השתנת חד ב 10 דנב ... החמות: om. O

5 Plane tree (*Platanus orientalis*); Rom. PWŠṬʾ: Its leaves and nuts are cold [and] dry; it is good for a burn if one pounds them in vinegar and applies this as a poultice. If one burns the rind in vinegar and uses it as a gargle, it is good for toothache.

6 Lees of wine; Rabb. Hebr. SMRY HYYN: It is hot; it abates and dissolves inflamed tumors when it is rubbed on them. Lees of vinegar do not heat; they calm (reduce) inflamed tumors when it is rubbed on them.

7 Soot: The [properties of] soot resulting from [the burning of substances] depends on the [kind of substances] it hails from. But any soot is hot and dry and its properties are those of the substance from which it hails.

8 Dragon's blood (lit., blood of the two brothers; red resin derived from *Dracaena draco*); Rom. ŠNG DRʾGYN: It is cold; it constipates the bowels and closes up fresh wounds.

9 Cantharides (Spanish flies); Rom. QNTRYDŠ; Rabb. Heb. MʾYRWT: They are hot [and] sharp; they are good for mange; if one ingests a large quantity they cause an ulcer in the urinary bladder and bleeding and are possibly fatal; a small dosis stimulates diuresis.

10 "Horse-tail" (a variety of *Equisetum*); [Hebr.] ZNB HSWS; Rom. QWDʾ DQʾBL: It is cold [and] good for diarrhea, hemoptysis, and inflamed tumors.

11 Gold; [Hebr.] ZHB; Rom. ʾWR: It is good for palpitations of the heart and for anxiety.

---

5 "Plane tree" (DLB): Cf. IĞ 237. 6 "Lees of wine" (DRDY): Cf. SHS 1:178 (Dalet 17). ‖ "it abates and dissolves inflamed tumors when it is rubbed on them": "it dissolves inflamed tumors" O. 7 "Soot … from which it hails": Om. O. 8 "Dragon's blood" (DM ʾLʾKWYN): Cf. IĞ 1032; SHS 1:168 (Dalet 2). 9 "Cantharides (Spanish flies)" (DRʾRYḤ): Cf. SHS 1:311–312 (Mem 16); "Cantharides … diuresis": Om. O. 10 "'Horse-tail'" (DNB ʾLKYL): Cf. IĞ 501; SHS 1:199–200 (Zayin 4); "'Horse-tail' … tumors": Om. O. 11 "Gold" (DHB): Cf. SHS 1:155–156 (Gimel 15). ‖ "palpitations of the heart (heart burn)": Cf. Dalet 1 above. ‖ "anxiety": Cf. NM 4 s.v. השתוממות (forthcoming).

אות ההא

1 הלילג השחור ובלעז מירבולנש אינדיש וב״מ הלילקים הודיים: נאותים לטבעים כלם ולכל חולי ואין דבר בכלל יותר חשוב ולא יותר רב התועלת ממנו והוא ישלשל שלשול חלוש ויעבד האצטומכה ויועיל מן הטחורים.

2 הלילג אצפר: קר משלשל מרה כרכומית.

3 האל: חם יבש דק טוב לקרירות האצטומכה והכבד.

4 היוקסטידאס איבוקושטידום ויקרא זקן התיש: קר קובץ ראוי להרגילו כשיביא הצורך לעצור ולקבוץ.

5 היופאריקום ובלע׳ אנפסק או ארבה פורבאדה: חם דק פותח הסתומים.

אות הואו

1 וג: ⟨חם יבש⟩ טוב מן הרוחות העבות והטחול ⟨הקשה⟩ וכובד הלשון

2 ושמה: חמה קובצת תצביע השער ותמעיט השכחה.

---

1 נאותים לטבעים כלם ולכל חולי ואין דבר בכלל יותר חשוב ולא יותר רב התועלת ממנו: om. O ‖ ויעבד: يدبغ O ‖ הטחורים: והוא חם רך ממוצע פותח לסתומים מתיך הלחה הלבנה העבה והלחה התפלה ויש סגולה במוח ובחושים add. א 2 כרכומית: ופותח הסתומין ומכבה המרה ומעבד המרה (= האצטומכה) ויקרא בלעז מירבולנש סיטרינש וב״ח הלילקים כרכומיים add. א 3 האל: هيل بوا O 4 היוקסטידאס: emend. ed. היופסטידאם א ⟨...⟩ ב 5 דק: קר א

1 ⟨חם יבש⟩: حارّ يابس O ‖ והטחול ⟨הקשה⟩: الطحال الصلب O 2 ותמעיט השכחה: om. O

He

1 Black myrobalans, i.e., Indian myrobalans (*Terminalia horrida Stend*); Rom. MYRBWLNŠ ʾYNDYŠ; Rabb. Hebr. HLYLQYM HWDYYM: They are suitable (good) for all natures and for every disease. No [remedy] is more eminent and more useful than this one; it has a weak purgative [power]; it strengthens the stomach and is good for hemorrhoids.

2 Yellow myrobalan (*Terminalia citrina Roxb.*): It is cold [and] purges the yellow bile.

3 Cardamom (*Elettaria Cardamomum*): It is hot, dry, and fine; it is good for a cold stomach and liver.

4 "Goatsbeard" (*Tragopogon pratensis*, or *Tragopogon porrifolius*); ʾYBWQWŠṬYDWM; also called [Hebr.] ZQN HTYŠ: It is cold [and] astringent; one should use it in case it is necessary to use [retaining and astringent ingredients].

5 Hypericum; Rom. ʾNPSQ or ʾRBH PWRBʾDH: It is cold [and] fine; it opens obstructions.

Waw

1 Sweet flag (*Acorus calamus*): It is hot [and] dry [and] good for thick winds, hardness of the spleen, and heaviness of tongue.

2 Woad (*Isatis tinctoria*): It is hot and astringent; [it is good for] coloring the hair and for reducing forgetfulness.

---

1 "Black myrobalans" (HLYLG HŠḤWR): Cf. SHS 1:186 (He 8). ‖ "They are suitable (good) for all natures and for every disease. No [remedy] is more eminent and more useful than this one; it has a weak purgative [power]": Om. O. ‖ "strengthens the stomach" (יעבד האצסטומכה): Cf. Alef 22 above. 2 "Yellow myrobalan" (HLYLG ʾṢPR): Cf. SHS 1:184–185 (He 6). ‖ "bile": א adds, "it opens obstructions; it extinguishes [the heat of] the bile and strengthens the stomach and is called in Rom. MYRBWLNŠ and in Rabb. Hebr. HLYLQYM KRKWMYYM" (cf. SHS 1:184–185 [He 6]). 3 "Cardamom" (HʾL): Cf. IĞ 280. 4 "'Goatsbeard'" (HYWQSṬYDʾS): Cf. IĞ 501; SHS 1:360–361 (Samekh 12). See also Pe 17 below. 5 "Hypericum" (HYWPʾRYQWM): For its different species see DT 3:146; see also Pe 16 below.

1 "Sweet flag" (WG): Cf. IĞ 52. 2 "Woad (*Isatis tinctoria*)" (WŠMH) (Arab.: *wasma*): The Arab. term can also refer to "indigo" (*Indigofera tinctoria*); cf. IĞ 297. ‖ "and for reducing forgetfulness": Om. O.

אות הזין

1 זנגביל ובלע׳ זינגברי וב״ח זינגביל: חם יבש מעכל המאכל ומרפה המעים נאות לקרירות האצטומכה והכבד ולחשיכת הראות הבאה מצד הלחויות כשיאכל או כשיוכחל בו.

2 זראונד הוא שני מינים ארוכה ועגולה ובלעז ארישטולוגיאה לונגא וארישטולוגיא רדונדא: כל מיניו חמים פותחים הסתומים טובים מעקיצת העקרבים ומגירים דם הנדות ומוציאים העובר.

3 זופא בלעז איזופוש או איזוף: היבש ממנו הצומח מן הארץ חם יבש במעלת האזוב ינקה החזה והריאה ויועיל מן הרנפלי והשעול הישן וישלשל הלחה הלבנה ויוציא התולעים מן הבטן. אך הלח הרטוב ממנו אשר הוא לכלוך הצמר יתיך המורסות הגסות וכל שכן אשר תהיינה בצדי כיס מקוה המים והרחמים.

4 זרנבאד: חם יבש יתיך הרוחות ויועיל מעקיצת הרמשים.

5 זאג ובלעז ארגימנט או ויטרייול וב״ח קלקנתוס: חם יבש ינגב הגרב והסעפה ויפסיק רעיפת הדם כשינפחו ממנו בנחירים והגרת הדם ממכה ⟨כ⟩שינתן עליהם

6 זיבק ובלעז ארגינט ביב וב״מ כסף חי: כשיומת יהיה שורף וטוב לגרב ולכנים.

---

2 לונגא: emend. ed. לוגנא א || רדונדא: emend. ed. רדונא א 3 זופא: אופא א || מן הבטן om. O

4 הרמשים: جدّا add. O 5 זאג: אלחמר א add. || הגרב: الرطب add. O || והגרת הדם: emend. ed. ומהגרת הדם ב om. א 6 זיבק ... ולכנים: om. O

Zayin

1 Ginger (*Zingiber officinalis Roscoe*); Rom. ZYNGBRY; Rabb. Hebr. ZYNGBYL: It is hot [and dry]; it [is good for] the digestion of the food and it loosens the intestines; it is beneficial for coldness of the stomach and liver; and if one eats it or applies it as an eye-salve, it is good for the darkening of the vision caused by humors.

2 Birthwort (*Aristolochia longa, A. rotunda*); it consists of two kinds: long and round; Rom. ARYŠṬWLWGY'H LWNG' and ARYŠṬWLWGY' RDWND': All its species are hot; they open obstructions, are good for scorpion stings, promote menstruation, and expel the foetus.

3 ZWP'; Rom. 'YZWPWŠ or 'YZWP: The dry [variety] which grows from the earth is as hot [and] dry as 'ZWB: It cleanses the chest and lungs and is beneficial for asthma and chronic cough; it purges phlegm and expels worms from the belly. But moist *zūfā*, i.e., grease of wool, dissolves hard tumors, especially those that are in the region of the urinary bladder and womb.

4 Bitter ginger (shampoo ginger, *Zingiber zerumbet*): It is hot [and] dry; it dissolves winds and is good for the stings and bites of vermin.

5 Vitriol; Rom. 'RGYMNṬ or WYṬRYYWL; Rabb. Heb. QLQNTWS: It is hot [and] dry; it dries mange and cradle cap and stops a nosebleed when it is snuffed up the nose and [it stops] a bleeding caused by a blow when it is applied to that spot.

6 Quicksilver; Rom. 'RGYNṬ BYB; Rabb. Hebr. KSP ḤY: When it is mortified it burns and is good for mange and lice.

---

1 "Ginger" (ZNGBYL): Cf. IĞ 1027. 2 "Birthwort" (ZR'WND): Cf. IĞ 321; IT 30b, c. 3 "ZWP'" (*zūfā*): Arab. *zūfā* means 1) "hyssop" (*Hyssopus officinalis*) and 2) "grease of wool." In Arabic, the different meanings are generally distinguished by the adjective reading *zūfā raṭb* ("moist *zūfā*") for "grease of wool," and *zūfā yābis* ("dry *zūfā*") for "hyssop"; cf. SHS 1:174–175 (Dalet 10). ‖ Hebrew 'ZWB is "hyssop," not the *Hyssopus officinalis*, which does not grow in Palestine, but probably *Origanum maru* or *Majorana syriaca*; cf. SHS 1:92–93 (Alef 2). O reads: السعتر; i.e., "origan," *Origanum*. ‖ "from the belly": Om. O. 4 "Bitter ginger" (ZRNB'D): Cf. IĞ 206. 5 "Vitriol" (Z'G) ("red vitriol" א): Cf. IĞ 865; SHS 1:454–455 (Qof 11). ‖ "mange": Cf. O: "moist mange." 6 "Quicksilver" (ZYBQ): Cf. KM 692–697; "Quicksilver ... lice": Om. O. ‖ "KSP ḤY": Cf. BM 2467–2468.

7 זרניך ובלעז אורפימנט: כל מיני זרניך חמים שורפים מועילים מן הגרב והבהק ומדוה השועל והשעפה הלחה והעיפוש והאכול והכנה והרנפלי כשיקטירו בו ויסירו רשומי הדם המת מן ההכאה בשוטים.

8 זבד אלבחר ובלעז אשפומא דמר: כל מיניו חמים יבשים טובים לבהק והגרב ומדוה השועל.

9 זכוכית: יש לו סגולה יפרך בה החצץ המתילד בכיס מקוה המים ויסיר הילפת כשרוחצין בו הראש.

10 זרנב אלפלור דסנמומי וב״ח נץ של דרצין: חם יבש טוב לאצטומכה והכבד הקרים ומאמץ המעים.

11 זנגאר ובלעז ווירדיט וב״ח פרת נחשת: חם יבש אוכל הבשר ופותח המורסא הגסה.

12 זנגופר ובלעז וירמליון וב״מ ששר: חם יכנס אל הרטיות יועיל אל החבורות המעופשות תועלת גדולה והרוצה להרגילו צריך לשחקו ולזרותו על האיכולים כי הוא מנגבם ומנגב כל שחין מעופש.

---

7 שורפים: שרופים ב || ומדוה השועל om. O || והרנפלי והרנפיל ב || ויסירו: وإذا طلي به أذهب O
8 אשפומא דמר: זכוכית א || כל ... השועל: יש לו סגולה יפרך בה החצץ המתילד בכיס מקוה המים ויסיר הילפת כשרוחצין בו הראש א 9 זכוכית ... הראש: om. א || הילפת: الإبرية O 10 אלפלור: emend. ed. אלעפלור א || המעים: ובנוסחא אחרת טוב לגרב והבהק ומדוה השועל add. אב 11 יבש: om. O || ופותח המורסא הגסה: om. O || המורסא הגסה: המורסות הגסות ב 12 זנגופר: emend. ed. זנגפור אב || זנגופר ... שחין מעופש: om. O || ולזרותו: ולזכותו א

7 Arsenic; Rom. ʾWRPYMNṬ: All varieties of arsenic are hot and burning; they are useful for mange, *bahaq*, alopecia, moist cradle cap; putrefaction, corrosion, lice and asthma when they are applied as a fumigation. They remove the traces of dead blood resulting from flagellation.

8 ZBD ʾLBḤR (sea-foam); Rom. ʾŠPWMʾ DMR: All its varieties are hot [and] dry; they are good for *bahaq*, mange, and alopecia.

9 Glass: It has a specific property to pulverize stones that develop in the urinary bladder; it removes dandruff when the head is washed with it.

10 ZRNB; [Rom.] ʾLʿPLWR DSNMWMY; Rabb. Heb. NẒ ŠL DRẒYN: It is hot [and] dry; it is good for a cold stomach and cold liver; it constipates the bowels.

11 Verdigris; Rom. WWYRDYṬ; Rabb. Hebr. PRḤ NḤŠT: It is hot [and] dry; it corrodes the flesh and opens a hard tumor.

12 Cinnabar; Rom. WYRMLYWN; Rabb. Hebr. ŠŠR: It is hot; when it is put in a plaster it is very beneficial for putrid wounds. If you want to apply it, you should pulverize it and strew it on corroding sores because it dries them; it dries all putrid tumors.

---

7 "Arsenic" (ZRNYK): Cf. KM 658–664; SHS 1:353–354 (Samekh 2). || *Bahaq*: Arab. *bahaq* stands for Greek ἀλφός (cf. UW 97: "weisse Hautflecken"); Richard Durling, *A Dictionary of Medical Terms in Galen* (Leiden: Brill, 1993), p. 34, translates the Greek term as "dull-white leprosy"; for an extensive discussion of the different types of *bahaq*, see Ibn al-Jazzār, *Zād al musāfir wa-qūt al-ḥāḍir. Provisions for the Traveller and Nourishment for the Sedentary, Book 7* (7–30), ed. and trans. Gerrit Bos (Leiden: Brill, 2015), ch. 18, 1–3 (pp. 108–110). || "alopecia" (מדוה השועל): Cf. NM 2:14. || "They remove": Cf. O: "When rubbed [on the spot] they remove." 8 "ZBD ʾLBḤR" (= *zabad al-baḥr*): Arab. *zabad al-baḥr*, "sea foam," is the translation of Greek ἀλκυόνιον "bastard-sponge" (LS 67) and designates according to Dioscurides (5:118) "a mixture of sponges, algae and polypiers rejected by the sea" (DT 1:9 n. 3; M 141); cf. SHS 1:228 (Ḥet 33). || Cf. Zayin 7 above. 9 "dandruff" (ילפת): Cf. NM 2:12–13. 10 "ZRNB" (*zarnab*): The Arabic term has not yet been identified satisfactorily; cf. IĞ 317; SHS 1:434 (Ṣade 9). || א and ב add, "and following another version: It is good for mange, *bahaq* and alopecia." 11 "Verdigris" (ZNGʾR): Cf. KM 2:669–673; SHS 1:406–407 (Pe 11). || "and opens a hard tumor": Om. O. 12 "Cinnabar" (ZNGWPR): Cf. KM 2:677–683; SHS 1:500 (Shin 7); "ZNGPWR ... tumors": Om. O.

אות החית

1 חמאמא ובלעז אממו: חם יבש טוב לסתומי הכבד כשיהיו עם קור ומועיל למכאובי הרחמים ויכביד הראש ויגרום חוג.

2 חאשא: חם מועיל מחולשת הראות הבאה מצד הלחות כשכוחלין אותו או אוכלין ממנו וגורם מיחוש בראש והוא טוב אל הרינפלי ויוציא התולעים ויפיל העובר ועוזר על העיכול.

3 חב אלניל ובלע׳ גראנא דאינדי וב״ח גרגרי האיסטיס: ישלשל הליחה הלבנה ויועיל מן הצרעת והבהק הלבן אלא שהוא יצער וגורם אסטניסות ויקרא בלשון הגרי חב אלערוס.

4 חי אלעאלם ובלעז כובא קורבינא וב״ח חיי עולם: קר טוב למורסות החמות כשיטחו בו ומכבה שרפת האש והדשן כשיוטח בו.

5 חנטל ובלעז קולוקוינטידא וב״ח פקועות: חם יבש דק ישלשל ליחה לבנה עבה וינקה הראש ויועיל ממכאובי העצבים וגיד הנשה והפדגרא הקרה ומדוה הפיל.

6 חרמל: ⟨חם⟩ גורם שכרות וחוג ומעורר הקיא ומגיר השתן ודם הנדות.

---

1 חוג: ويصدع add. O 2 כשכוחלין אותו או אוכלין ממנו: إذا أكل O ‖ וגורם (וגורמים א) מיחוש בראש: om. O 3 אלניל: emend. ed. אלגיל אב ‖ הלבנה: بقوة add. O ‖ הצרעת: البرص O ‖ חב אלערוס: om. א 4 אלעאלם: אלעאלים א ‖ קר טוב למורסות החמות כשיטחו בו ומכבה שרפת האש והדשן כשיוטח בו: om. א ‖ כשיוטח בו: om. O 6 גורם ... חוג (= ويسدّر): ويسدّد O

Ḥet

1 ḤM’M’; Rom. ’MMW: It is hot [and] dry; it is beneficial for obstructions of the liver when these are accompanied by cold; it is good for pains in the uterus; it causes heaviness of the head and dizziness (stupefaction).

2 Ḥ’Š’: It is hot [and] beneficial for weakness of vision caused by moisture when it is applied as an eye-salve or when it is eaten; it causes headache; it is good for asthma; it expels worms, causes a miscarriage, and helps the digestion.

3 “Seed of indigo”; Rom. GR’N’ D’YNDY; Rabb. Heb. GRGRY H’YSṬYS: It purges the phlegm and is beneficial for leprosy and white *bahaq*, but it causes distress and nausea. In Arabic it is called ḤB ’L-‘RWS.

4 “Houseleek” (*Sempervivum arboreum*, or *Sempervivum tectorum*); Rom. KWB’ QWRBYN’; Rabb. Hebr. ḤYY ‘WLM: It is cold [and] good for inflamed tumors, burns, and ophthalmia when it is rubbed on them.

5 Colocynth (*Citrullus colocynthis*); Rom. QWLWQWYNṬYD’; Rabb. Heb. PQW‘WT: It is hot, dry, [and] fine; it purges thick phlegm, cleanses the head, and is beneficial for painful nerves (neuralgia), ischias, cold podagra, and elephantiasis.

6 Harmel (*Peganum harmala*): [It is hot]; it intoxicates, and causes dizziness; it makes the urine and menstual blood flow.

---

1 “ḤM’M’” (Arab. *ḥamāmā*): Possibly South Indian Treebine, *Cissus vitiginea* (now known as *Cissus angulata*); cf. SP 252; Dietrich (DT 1:12) remarks that it is a plant belonging to the Vitiginea family, but that an exact identification is impossible. ‖ “dizziness (stupefaction)”: “and headache” add. O. 2 “Ḥ’Š’”: A species of thyme or mint; cf. IĞ 157; SHS 1:455–456 (Qof 13). ‖ “when it is applied as an eye-salve or”: Om. O. ‖ “it causes headache”: Om. O. 3 “‘Seed of indigo’”: In Arabic, it stands for the seed of a blue variety of morning glory (ivy-leaved morning glory, *Ipomoea nil*); cf. IĞ 382. ‖ for leprosy; cf. O “baraṣ”: This skin disease has two varieties, white and black, which are sometimes summarized under the general term *baraṣ*. The white variety is perhaps identical with *Sklerodermia circumscripta*, while the black variety may be *Psoriasis vulgaris* or *Ichhthyosis vulgaris*; cf. Ibn al-Jazzār, *Zād al musāfir wa-qūt al-ḥāḍir. Provisions for the Traveller and Nourishment for the Sedentary, Book 7* (7–30), ed. and trans. Bos p. 108, n. 195. ‖ “white *bahaq*”: Cf. Zayin 7 above. ‖ “nausea”: Cf. Bet 10 above. ‖ “ḤB ’l-‘RWS” (حبّ العروس): The identification of ḤB ’L-‘RWS as “seed of indigo” could not be retrieved. It features as another term for “cubeb,” next to *kabāba* in M 194. 4 “Houseleek” (ḤY ’L‘’LM): Cf. IĞ 36; SHS 1:211 (Ḥet 4). ‖ “ophthalmia” (דשן): Cf. NM 2:11. 5 “Colocynth” (ḤNZL): Cf. IĞ 284; SHS 1: 220–221 (Ḥet 20). 6 “Harmel” (ḤRML): Cf. IĞ 31, 131; SHS 1:504 (Shin 14). ‖ “causes dizziness” (גורם חוג): Cf. NM 2:12.

7 חסך ובלעז טריבולוס מרינוש או אשפונגא מרי וב״מ שמיר: חם יפרך החצץ כשישתו ממנו ויוסיף בתאות המשגל ויתיר עצירת השתן.

8 חב אלרשאד ובלעז נשטורש וב״ח שחלים: חם יבש רע לאצטומכה יועיל מהלחויות והרוחות העבות ויעורר תאות המשגל ויהרוג העובר במעי אמו ויש אומרים שהוא חם מאד מחמם האצטומכה והכבד ומרפה המעים ומוציא מהם התולעים ומעורר התאוה ומועיל מן הרנפלי ועובי הטחול.

9 חנא ובלעז אלקינא: מנעימה הגוף טובה לשחין הפה הנקרא בלשון הגרי קלאע ושרפת האש ולריח הטרכסיד.

10 חצץ ובלע׳ ליסיאום: בינוני בחום ובקור יועיל למורסות החמות בעין כשיוטח בו עליהם ולמורסות התפוחות ויועיל מן החניקה כשיתגרגרו בו ומן השחין בפה.

11 חדיד ובלעז פירי וב״מ ברזל: סיגיו מחזקים האצטומ׳ ומפסיקים דם הטחורים והמים המכניס בו הברזל מעוררים תאות המשגל ומסירים עובי הטחול.

---

7 חסך: חסכך א || טריבולוס: .emend. ed טריבולום א אטריפל ב || חם: بارد O 8 חב אלרשאד: حرف O חב ... הטחול: حارّ جدّا مسخن للمعدة والكبد ملين للبطن يخرج الدود ويحرّك شهوة الباه وينّقي الرئة وينفع من الربو وغلظ الطحال ويسقط الأجنّة O || מהלחויות: מהלחות ב || במעי: בבטן ב 9 מנעימה הגוף: .om O || ולריח הטרכסיד: .om O 10 יועיל למורסות החמות ... ולמורסות התפוחות: نافع للأورام الرخوة الرهلة وللأورام الحارّة O 11 סיגיו: סוגיו א

7 Caltrops (*Tribulus terrestris*); Rom. ṬRYBWLWS MRYNWŠ or ʾŠPWNGʾ MRY; Rabb. Hebr. ŠMYR: It is hot; when it is ingested it pulverizes stones, increases the libido, and cures dysuria.

8 Seed of garden cress (*Lepidum sativum*); Rom. NŠṬWRŠ; Rabb. Hebr. ŠḤLYM: It is hot [and] dry; it is bad for the stomach [and] beneficial for thick humors and winds; it arouses the sexual lust and kills the foetus in the womb of the mother. According to some, it is very hot; it heats the stomach and the liver, loosens the intestines, expels intestinal worms, whets the appetite, and is useful for asthma and thickness of the spleen (enlarged spleen).

9 Henna (*Lawsonia inermis*); Rom. ʾLQYNʾ: It fattens the body; it is good for ulcers in the mouth, which are called "qilāʿ" in Arabic, for burns, and for the smell of ṬRKSYD.

10 Buckthorn (*Lycium sp*); Rom. LYSYʾWM: It is moderate in heat and cold; it is beneficial for flabby tumors and inflammations in the eyes when it is rubbed on them; it is beneficial for angina and for ulcers in the mouth when it is used as a gargle.

11 Iron; Rom. PYRY; Rabb. Hebr. BRZL: [Iron] dross strengthens the stomach and stops hemorrhoidal bleedings; water mixed with iron arouses sexual lust and reduces thickness of the spleen (enlarged spleen).

---

7 "Caltrops" (ḤSK): Cf. IĞ 229; SHS 1:497 (Shin 4). ‖ "hot": "cold" O. 8 "Seed of garden cress" (ḤB ʾLRŠʾD): Cf. IĞ 1030; SHS 1:503 (Shin 12). ‖ "It is hot ... spleen": "It is very hot [and] heats the stomach and the liver, relieves the bowels, expels worms, stimulates sexual lust, cleanses the lungs, is beneficial for asthma and thickness of the spleen, and causes a miscarriage" O. 9 "Henna" (ḤNʾ): Cf. SHS 1:275 (Kaf 20). ‖ "It fattens" (מנעימה): The Hebrew term stands for Arab. خصب, which features in al-Zahrāwī, *Kitāb al-taṣrīf*, and is translated by Shem Tov as הנעים; cf. NM 4, s.v. נעם (forthcoming): וינעים הגופים הבריאים וכל שכן כשיהיה מן החטה האדומה הכבדה (It [i.e, broth prepared from wheat flour] fattens the body, especially that prepared from heavy red wheat); "It fattens the body": Om. O. ‖ "qilāʿ": I.e., aphthae. ‖ "and for the smell of ṬRKSYD": Om. O. ‖ "ṬRKSYD": I.e., "binding cement; stony and rocky lime"; the Geonim identified it as "ceruse"; cf. SHS 1:241–242 (Ṭet 3). 10 "Buckthorn" (ḤṢṢ): Cf. IĞ 512; IT, Lamed 10. 11 "Iron" (ḤDYD): Cf. SHS 1:236 (Ḥet 49).

אות הטית

1 טוראתית ובלעז רושא קנינא וב״מ זקן תיש: קר יבש טוב לקיא ולשלשול ואמרו שהוא מאמץ המעים.

2 טין מכתום ובלע׳ בול שגלאטום וב״ח טיט חתום הארמי: טוב לרקיקת הדם ולשלשולו והנאכל ממנו אטמים בכבד וגורם הפסד מזג אלא שהוא מחזק פי האצטומכה ויסיר ממנה זוהמת המטעם המזוהם וישקיט אסטניסות וייטיב הנפש.

3 טין אלבולין הוא הטיט הרומיי: מאמץ המעים ומועיל מרקיקת הדם והוא במקום התותיא ויחבש האברים הנשברים.

4 טרפא ובלע׳ טמריסי: קר יבש והתחבושת העשוי מעליו תועיל לצמחים התפוחים ⟨...⟩ והמגמע במים נתבשלו בו העלים יכלכל(?) הטחול ואם יעשה משרש טני וישתה בו מים או יין או אשירוב אסיטוס בהתמדה יסיר נפח הטחול ואם יעשה משרש ממנו בין ידי אשר מצאם תונבא יועיל תועלת מבוארת וישבור נזק השחין הנקרא בלשונם גרב וכשימשוך ריחו בעל הזיכום יסירנו.

---

1 טוב: من الحمّى الحادّة والعطش و– add. O || ואמרו שהוא מאמץ המעים: وللخفقان والقلاع O 2 בול: emend. ed. שגבול א || הארמי: وطين أرمني O || לרקיקת: לרקיקות א || וישקיט: ויסיר א || וייטיב הנפש: om. O 3 טין ... הנשברים: om. O || אלבולין: אלכולין ב 4 טרפא: טורפא א || והתחבושת העשוי: והתחבושות העשויים א || ⟨...⟩: والتمضمض بطبيخه يسكن وجع الأسنان add. O || והמגמע ... הטחול: وإن شرب الشراب الذي يطبخ فبه ورقه أذبل الطحال O || יסירנו: emend. ed. יסדירנו? א

Ṭet

1 Maltese mushroom (*Cynomorium coccineum*); Rom. RWŠʾ QNYNʾ; Rabb. Hebr. ZQN TYŠ: It is cold [and] dry; it is good for vomiting and for diarrhea; it is said that it constipates the bowels.

2 Terra sigillata (or Lemnian earth); Rom. BWL ŠGLʾṬWM; Rabb. Hebr. ṬYṬ ḤTWM and Armenian earth: It is good for hemoptysis and bloody diarrhea; if one eats from it, it causes obstructions of the liver and corruption of the temperament, [but] it strengthens the cardia of the stomach, removes the stench of spoilt food from it, and alleviates nausea and is good for the soul.

3 ṬYN ʾL-BWLYN; i.e., Romaic clay: It constipates the bowels, is good for hemoptysis and is a [good] substitute for tutty and [is good for] setting broken limbs.

4 French tamarisk (different species of Tamaricaceae; perhaps French tamarisk [*Tamarix gallica*]); Rom. ṬMRYSY: It is cold [and] dry; a plaster prepared from its leaves is beneficial for soft tumors; a gargle prepared from a decoction of it alleviates toothache; if one sips a decoction of its leaves it reduces an [enlarged] spleen; and if one prepares from its roots a drinking cup (?) and constantly drinks water or wine or oxymel from it, it reduces a swollen spleen (enlarged spleen). And if [some] of its roots are put in the hands of someone affected by numbness, it is clearly beneficial for him. It counteracts the harm [caused by] the tumor called "ǧarab" (mange) [in Arabic]. If someone suffering from a catarrh inhales its smell, he will be cured.

---

1 "Maltese mushroom": Cf. IĞ 276, 416; SHS 1:197–198 (Zayin 2). ‖ Arab. *ṭarāṯīṯ* is also identified as "goat's beard" (*Tragopogon porrifolius*, or *Tragopogon pratensis*); cf. IĞ 276. ‖ "It is good for vomiting": "It is good for acute fever, thirst and vomiting" O. ‖ "it is said that it constipates the bowels": "and for palpitations and aphthae" O. 2 "Terra sigillata (or Lemnian earth)" (ṬYN MKTWM): Cf. SHS 1:239–240 (Ṭet 1). ‖ "and Armenian earth" (cf. M 172): Translated after O. Shem Tov reads: "Aramaic" or "Syrian." ‖ "nausea": Cf. Bet 10 above. ‖ "and is good for the soul": Om O. 3 "ṬYN ʾL-BWLYN; i.e., Romaic clay: It confines the bowels, is good for hemoptysis and is a [good] substitute for tutty and [is good for] setting broken limbs": Om. O. 4 "French tamarisk" (ṬRPʾ): Cf. IĞ 72; SP 470; IT, Tav 2. ‖ "a gargle prepared from a decoction of it alleviates toothache": Translated following O. ‖ "if one sips a decoction of its leaves it an [enlarged] spleen; and if one prepares from its roots a drinking cup (?) and constantly drinks water or wine or oxymel from it, it reduces a swollen spleen (enlarged spleen)": "if one drinks a decoction of its leaves it reduces a swollen spleen" O. ‖ "reduces": Translated after Arab. أذبل. ‖ "drinking cup" (*ṭani*): Cf. SHS 1:242 (Ṭet 4). ‖ "oxymel" (אשירוב אסיטוס; read אישרוב אסיטוס) stands for Arab. سكنجبين (oxymel); cf. NM 4, s.v. אישרוב אסיטוס (forthcoming). ‖ "numbness" (תונבא): Cf. NM 1:120. ‖ "catarrh" (זיכום): Cf. NM 1:89.

5 טבאשיר ובלעז אשפודיאום: קר יבש מועיל מן הקדחת החדה והצמא והשלשול והאסטניסות והשחין הנקרא אלקלאע.

6 טחלב ובלעז לינטילאה או לינטילולא שעל פני המים: קר טוב למורסות החמות כשיחובש בו.

אות היוד

1 יברוח ובלעז מנדרגולא: קר מקדיר ואם ישקוהו ביין משכר ואם ישקוהו בסמים ישקיט המכאובים ואם ירבו ממנו ימית.

2 יתוע ובלעז טיטמאל או לשושקלי: מיניו רבים וכולם חמים משלשלים ומקיאים ומשחינים הגוף.

3 ינבות: קר יבש יועיל לשלשול טוב לירקון כשישתה אדם ממימיו.

אות הכף

1 כמאפיטוס: חם טוב לעצירת השתן והירקון וגיד הנשה.

2 כנדס ובלעז כונדוס וב״מ קנינא: ⟨חם⟩ יש לו כח חזק ישלשל ויגרום הצמא.

---

5 קר יבש מועיל: = بارد يابس O[1] || מן ... אלקלאע: om. O || אלקלאע: emend. ed. אלקלאג א

1 כמאפיטוס: emend. ed. כיטום א כיטור ב كمافيطوس O

5 Tabasheer; Rom. ʾŠPWDYWM: It is cold [and] dry [and] beneficial for acute fever, thirst, diarrhea, nausea, and the ulceration called "qilāʿ" (aphthae).

6 Duckweed (*Lemna minor*); Rom. LYNṬYLʾH or LYNṬYLWLʾ, which [floats] on the water: It is cold [and] good for inflamed tumors when it is applied as a poultice.

Yod

1 Mandrake (*Mandragora officinarum* and Var.); Rom. MNDRGWLʾ: It is cold [and] narcotic; if it is administered in wine it has an intoxicating effect, and if it is administered with [other] drugs it alleviates pains, but if one takes too much it is fatal.

2 Spurge; Rom. ṬYṬMʾL or LŠWŠQLY: It has many species; all of them are hot and have a purgative, emetic, and ulcerating effect on the body.

3 Stinking bean trefoil (*Anagyris foetida*): It is cold [and] dry; when one drinks its juice it is beneficial for diarrhea and jaundice.

Kaf

1 Ground pine (yellow bugle) (*Ajuga chamaepitys*): It is hot [and] good for dysuria, jaundice, and ischias.

2 Sneezewort (*Achillea ptarmica*); Rom. KWNDWS; Rabb. Hebr. QNYNʾ: It is hot and very strong; it purges and causes thirst.

---

5 "Tabasheer" (ṬBʾŠYR): I.e., a white substance obtained from the nodal joints of bamboo (*Bambusa bambos*); cf. IĞ 904. || "nausea": Cf. Bet 10 above. 6 "Duckweed" (ṬḤLB): IĞ 708; SHS 1:377–378 (Ayin 2).

1 "Mandrake" (YBRWḤ): Cf. IĞ 426; SHS 1:169 (Dalet 3). || "narcotic": Cf. Bet 2 above. 2 "Spurge" (YTWʿ): A generic name of plants from the spurge family (*Euphorbia sp.*); cf. IĞ 425; SHS 1:509 (Shin 22). 3 "Stinking bean trefoil" (YNBWT): Cf. IĞ 427.

1 "Ground pine (yellow bugle)" (KMʾPYṬWS): Cf. IĞ 458. 2 "Sneezewort" (KNDS): The Arabic term can also refer to soapwort, fuller's herb (*Saponaria officinalis*), and gypsophila (species of gypsophila), the various roots of which contain saponin; cf. IĞ 82; SHS 1:213 (Ḥet 7). || Hebr. QNYNʾ is perhaps a corruption of ḤNYNʾ; cf. SHS 1:213 (Ḥet 7).

3 כזמאזך ובלע׳ גראנא דטמריס: קר מעכב הוסת ויאמץ המעים וישקיט הדם טוב למי שיתאכל מן השנים ושיתנועע מהם.

4 כהרבא ובלעז קקברי: קר יבש טוב להגרת הדם מן הנדות והטחורים ורקיקת הדם והשלשול יועיל מדפיקת הלב.

5 כמאדריוס ובלעז כאמידריוש וב״מ בטנים של ארץ: חם פותח הסתומים ויסיר עובי הטחול והירקון טוב לאפר העין ומכאובה.

6 כסילה: חם יבש יחמם הגוף טוב לאצטומכה.

7 כילדארוא: חם רך יוציא התולעים הנקראים גרגרי הדלועים שורף מצמיח ותועיל הטיחה בו מן הגרב.

8 כרם אלשראב: הדך זלזליו ועליו ויחבוש בהם ⟨המורסות⟩ החמים והראש אשר יש לה מיחוש יועילו והדך זלזליו וישתה מימיהם יפסיקו הקיא ויאמצו המעים.

9 כנדר ובלעז אנשנש לבונה: חם יבש מצמיח בשר בשחין ויפסיק השלשול והמרבה ממנו ישרוף הדם ויתן בינה עד שאפשר שיגרום למרגילו שטות.

10 כבאבה ובלע׳ קובבש: חם יפתח הסיתומים וינקה מעברי השתן ויזכך הגרון ויאמץ המעים.

---

3 כזמאזך: emend. ed. כרמאזך אב ‖ קר: يابس add. O ‖ מעכב: הדם ב מעכב ... הדם: يحبس البطن وسيلان الدم add. O ‖ וישקיט הדם טוב למי שיתאכל מן השנים: om. ב ‖ טוב: emend. ed. הטוב א ‖ ושיתנועע מהם: om. א 5 כמאדריוס: חם רד add. א ‖ טוב לאפר העין ומכאובה: om. O 6 יחמם: יחם ב يسمن O 7 כילדארוא: كِلدَاروة O ‖ רד: רע ב om. O ‖ שורף מצמיח ותועיל הטיחה בו מן הגרב om. O 8 ⟨המורסות⟩: الأورام O 9 השלשול: om. א والقيء add. O ‖ ישרוף: יפסיק א ‖ שטות: وسواس O 10 מעברי: מעבר א مجاري O

3 Gallnut of the tamarisk (*Tamarix articulata Vahl* [*Tamarix orientalis Forsk.*]); Rom. GR’N’ DṬMRYS: It is cold; it stops [excessive] menstruation, constipates the bowels, and stops a bleeding; it is good for corrosion and movement of the teeth.

4 Amber; Rom. QQBRY: It is cold [and] dry; it is good for [excessive] menstrual bleeding, hemorrhoids, hemoptysis, and diarrhea, [and] beneficial for palpitations of the heart.

5 Germander (*Teucrium chamaedrys*); Rom. K’MYDRYWŠ; Rabb. Heb. BṬNYM ŠL ’RṢ: It is hot; it opens obstructions, reduces thickness of the spleen (enlarged spleen), and cures jaundice; it is good for ophthalmia and pain in the eyes.

6 KSYLH (= *kissīlā*): It is hot [and] dry; it heats the body and is good for the stomach.

7 Fern (*Dryopteris filix mas* [*L.*] *Schott* and Var.): It is hot [and] fine; it expels tapeworms; it burns, stimulates the growth, and it is beneficial for mange when it is rubbed on it.

8 Vine: If you pound its tendrils and leaves and apply this as a poultice to inflamed tumors and to the head [of someone suffering from] headache, it will be beneficial. And if you pound its tendrils and drink its juice, it stops vomiting and constipates the bowels.

9 Frankincense (the resin of diverse species of the genus *Boswellia sp.*); Rom. ’NŠNŠ [Rabb. Hebr.] LBWNH: It is hot [and] dry; it regenerates the flesh in an ulcer and stops diarrhea; if one takes an overdose, it burns the blood; it sharpens the intellect, but it may cause delusion (delirium).

10 Cubeb pepper (fruit of *Piper cubeba*); Rom. QWBBŠ: It is hot; it opens the obstructions, cleanses the urethra and the throat, and constipates the bowels.

---

3 “Gallnut of the tamarisk” (KZM’ZK): Cf. IĞ 456. || “cold”: “[and] dry” add. O. 4 “Amber” (KHRB’): Cf. WKAS 1:406. || “palpitations of the heart”: Cf. Dalet 1 above. 5 “Germander”: Cf. SHS 1:146 (Bet 30). || “it is good for ophthalmia and pain in the eyes”: Om. O. || “ophthalmia”: Cf. Alef 17 above. 6 “*kissīla*”: The identity of this plant is unknown; cf. IBF 1931; D 1:468. || “heats”: “fattens” O. 7 “Fern” (KYLD’RW’): Persian كيلدارو; cf. IBF 1995: “Le nom persan signifie à la lettre ‘remède du Guilân;’” SC 1109a: “Name of a certain medicinal wood, black without and green within, found on the shores of the Caspian Sea.” || “fine”: Om. O. || “tapeworms” (גרגרי הדלועים): Cf. NM 2:11. || “it burns, stimulates the growth and it is beneficial for mange when it is rubbed on it”: Om. O. 8 “Vine” (KRM ’LŠR’B): Lit., “the vine (*Vitis vinifera*) that produces wine.” 9 “Frankincense” (KNDR): Cf. IĞ 252. || “diarrhea”: “and vomiting” add. O. || “delusion (delirium)” (שטות): Cf. Bet 12 above; “if someone takes it” add. אב. 10 “Cubeb pepper” (KB’BH): Cf. IĞ 490.

11 כברית ובלעז שופרי וב״מ גופרית: חמים דקים ינתנו עם התריאק או שתן נער על עקיצת העקרבים ועל עקיצת הרמשים כולם. הוא שלשה מינים כרכומיי ואדום ולבן והכרכומי והלבן יועילו מארס הרמשים כששוחקים אותם וזורים אותם עליהם והשותה מהם משקל שתי גרות יועילו והשוחק אותם וילוש אותם בחומץ ויטיח בהם על הצרעת והספחת והחכוך יסירו אותם.

12 ברכידס(?): יש בו חמיצות ולחות והוא מסכסך תאות המשגל ומשמין

13 כרבק: השחור ישלשל המרה השחורה והלבן יעורר הקיא ושתייתו סכנה גדולה.

14 כבת אלחדיד: יחזק האצטומכה ויפסיק דם הטחורים והמים המכבים בהם הברזל המחומם היטב מעוררים תאות המשגל וידלדלו כשישתו.

15 כטמי ובלעז מירקא או קטאפוסיא: חם טוב אל הירקון והפלג ומרכך כל כבד גס כשיחובש בו.

16 כרדל ובלעז ארגוה או שינבא: חם יחתך הליחה הלבנה כשיתן ממנו בנחירים ויוציא התולעים ויבשל המורסות.

---

11 שופרי: emend. ed. שובפרי א ‖ גופרית: מיניו כולם ב add. ‖ חמים ... יסירו אותם: محرق ينفع من الجرب إذا طلي به ومن الربو إذا شرب O ‖ והספחת: והגרב ב add. 12 ברכידס(?) ... ומשמין: om. O ‖ המשגל: ולחות א add. 13 המרה השחורה: om. O ‖ הקיא: بقوة قوية O add. 14 כבת ... כשישתו: om. O ‖ כשישתו: כשישתה ב 15 כטמי ... כשיחובש בו: om. ב ‖ חם ... בו: حارّ باعتدال يلين الأورام ويسكن الأوجاع وبزره يقلع البهق إذا طلي بخلّ في الشمس وينفع من حرقة البول O 16 כשיתן ממנו בנחירים: כשיתן ממנו ⟨...⟩ ב إذا تحنّك به O ‖ ויבשל המורסות: מהמורסות א ‖ המורסות: כרוע: חם טוב אל הדרקון והפלג ומרכך כל דבר גס כשיחובש בו ב add.

11 Sulphur; Rom. ŠWPRY; Rabb. Hebr. GWPRYT: It is hot [and] fine; [it is beneficial when] it is put with the theriac or the urine of a child on the stings of scorpions and of all vermin. It consists of three varieties: yellow, red, and white. The yellow and white varieties are beneficial for the poison of vermin when they are pulverized and strewn on the [spot of the sting or bite]. If someone drinks a dose of two carob seeds of [these varieties], it is beneficial for him. If they are pulverized, kneaded with vinegar, and rubbed on [spots affected by] leprosy, eczema, and itching, they will cure them.

12 KRKYDS(?): It has acidity and moisture; it stimulates the sexual lust and fattens.

13 Hellebore (i.e., black hellebore [*Helleborus niger*] or white hellebore [*Veratrum album* and Var.]): The black [variety] purges the black bile and the white [variety] induces vomiting and its ingestion is very dangerous.

14 Dross or rust of iron: It strengthens the stomach and stops hemorrhoidal bleeding; the water in which very hot iron [dross] has been quenched arouses sexual lust. It has a thinning (emaciating) effect when it is ingested.

15 Marshmallow (*Althaea officinalis*); Rom. MYRQ' or QṬ'PWSY': It is hot [and] good for jaundice and hemiplegia; it softens all hard livers when it is applied as a poultice.

16 Black mustard (*Brassica nigra*); Rom. 'RGWH or ŠYNB': It is hot; it dissolves the phlegm when it is chewed and then rubbed on the palate; it expels worms and ripens tumors.

---

11 "Sulphur" (KBRYT): Cf. SHS 1:152 (Gimel 11). ‖ "it … they will cure them": "when it is burnt and rubbed [on a spot affected by] mange, it is beneficial for it; [it is also good for] asthma if it is ingested" O. ‖ "theriac": A confection originally given as an antidote to snakebite and occasionally later as a general tonic. ‖ "eczema" (ספחת): The same Hebrew term features in Shem Tov's *Sefer ha-Shimmush* for Arab. قوباء (cf. NM 4, s.v. ספחת; forthcoming). 12 "KRKYDS(?)": This term could not be identified; "KRKYDS(?) … fattens": Om. O. 13 "Hellebore" (KRBQ): Cf. IĞ 1048; DT 4:137. ‖ "the black bile": Om. O. ‖ "induces vomiting": "is a strong vomitive" O. 14 "Dross or rust of iron" (KBT 'LḤDYD): Cf. KM 1:545–548; "Dross … ingested": Om. O. 15 "Marshmallow" (KṬMY): Cf. IĞ 1059; SHS 1:214 (Ḥet 9); "Marshmallow … poultice": Om. ב; "it is moderately hot; if softens hard tumors and alleviates pains; its seed cures (lit., exterminates) *bahaq* (see Zayin 7 above) when it is applied with vinegar as a poultice in the sun; it is also useful for burning urine" O. 16 "Black mustard" (KRDL): Cf. M 400. ‖ "when it is chewed and then rubbed on the palate": Translated after O. Shem Tov (א) reads, "when it is put in the nose." ‖ "tumors": "Castor-oil plant (*Ricinus communis*): It is hot and good for guinea-worms(?), hemiplegia and all indurations when it is applied as a poultice [to the spot]" add. ב.

17 כיארשנבר ובלעז קאשיפשטולא: מרכך הבטן ויאות לכל טבע ויועיל ממורסות הכסלים.

18 כמיר ובלעז לויאמי וב״ח שאור קמח חטה: טוב לכאב כף הרגל כשיחובש בו והוא מצמק הצמחים.

אות הלמד

1 לסאן אלחמל ובלעז פלנטאגי ובלשון חכמי׳ לשון טלה: קר טוב למורסות החמות ושרפת האש כשיחובש בו ולכאב האוזן החמה ויועיל זרעו לשחין המעים.

2 לך ובלעז לאקא: חם טוב ממכאובי הכבד והשקוי.

3 לסאן אלתור ובלעז לנגא בובינא וב״מ לשון השור: מועיל מתמהון לבב ומן דפיקת הלב ומהשחין הנקרא קלאע.

4 לוז מר וב״מ שקדים מרים: חם פותח הסתומים טוב לרנפלי ולחצץ הכליות וכיס מקוה המים.

5 לולו ובלע׳ גומאש או מרגרידש או פורלש וב״מ בדולח: קר יבש דק מנגב לחות העין ואם יעורב בסמי הכסלים יהיה מועיל וטוב.

6 לוף ובלעז שרפנטינא: חם פותח הסתומים יעורר תאות המשגל ויועיל לרנפלי הישן ומצמיח הבשר.

---

17 הכסלים: الحشا O 18 מצמק: منضج O

3 אלתור: אלתנר א 4 לוז ... המים: om. O 5 לולו: לולג א לולו ... וטוב: om. O ‖ וב״מ: קר א add. ‖ יעורב: יעורר ב 6 ומצמיח הבשר: om. O

17 Indian laburnum (*Cassia fistula*); Rom. Q'ŠYPŠṬWL': It softens the stools, is fitting for all natures (constitutions), and is beneficial for tumors in the entrails.

18 Yeast (KMYR); Rom. LWY'MY; Rabb. Hebr. Š'WR (leaven) from QMḤ ḤṬH (flour of wheat): It is good for pain in the sole of the foot when it is applied as a poultice [to the spot]; it shrinks abscesses.

Lamed

1 Plantain (*Plantago major*); Rom. PLNṬ'ĞY; Rabb. Hebr. LŠWN ṬLH: It is cold [and] good for inflamed tumors, burns, and hot ear pain when it is applied as a poultice [to the spot]; its seed is beneficial for intestinal ulcers.

2 Lac (shellac, from *Coccus lacca*); Rom. L'Q': It is hot [and] good for liver pains and dropsy.

3 Bugloss (*Anchusa officinalis*); Rom. LNG' BWBYN'; Rabb. Hebr. LŠWN HŠWR: It is beneficial for anxiety, for palpitations of the heart (heart burn), and for the ulceration called "qilā'" (aphthae).

4 Bitter almonds; Rabb. Hebr. ŠQDYM MRYM: They are hot; they open obstructions; they are good for asthma, for stones in the kidneys and urinary bladder.

5 Pearls; Rom. GWM'Š or MRGRYDŠ or PWRLŠ; Rabb. Hebr. BDWLḤ: They are cold, dry, [and] fine; they dry the moisture in the eyes, and if they are mixed with remedies for the inward parts of the body they are useful and good.

6 LWP (various species of arum [*Arum sp.*] and other plants); Rom. ŠRPNṬYN': It is hot; it opens obstructions, arouses sexual lust, is beneficial for chronic asthma, and regenerates flesh.

---

17 "Indian laburnum (KY'RŠNBR); Rom. Q'ŠYPŠṬWL'": Cf. IĞ 875; IT Qof 20. ‖ "entrails": As a rule, Shem Tov translates the Arabic حشاء as כסלים, which has the regular meaning of "loins"; cf. NM 4, s.v. כסל (forthcoming). 18 "shrinks": "ripens" O.

1 "Plantain (LS'N 'LḤML); Rom. PLNṬ'ĞY; Rabb. Hebr. LŠWN ṬLH": Cf. IĞ 507; SHS 1: 290–291 (Lamed 12). 2 "Lac" (LK): Cf. WKAS 2:1241b–1242a. 3 "Bugloss (LS'N 'LTWR); Rom. LNG' BWBYN'; Rabb. Hebr. LŠWN HŠWR": Cf. SHS 1:292 (Lamed 15). ‖ "palpitations of the heart (heart burn)": Cf. Dalet 1 above. 4 "Bitter almonds" (LWZ MR): Cf. IĞ 555; "Bitter ... bladder": Om. O. 5 "Pearls" (LWLW): Cf. WKAS 2,1:45–49; "Pearls ... good": Om. O. ‖ "BDWLḤ": Cf. JD 139. ‖ "inward parts of the body": Cf. Alef 17 above and NM 4, s.v. כסל (forthcoming). 6 "LWP" (= *lūf*): Cf. IĞ 504. ‖ "and regenerates flesh": Om. O.

7 לסאן אלעצאפיר ובלע׳ לנגא אויש וב״מ לשון צפור: יוסיף בשכבת הזרע ותאות המשגל ויפתח הסתומים ויועיל מדפיקת הלב.

אות המם

1 משכטראמשיר: חם מגיר השתן ודם הנדות.
2 מו ובלע׳ מוו: חם מועיל מעכוב השתן כשישתה ויחובש על הזקן התחתון.
3 מצטכי ובלעז משתיק: ⟨חם⟩ מחזק האצטומכה והכבד.
4 מקל אליהודי ובלע׳ בדליום גימיניס: ממסמס המורסות הגסות וטוב לטחורים.
5 מאהזהרה: ויקרא בלעז פאירי איננס פיל ובל״ח אבטרם הבן ⟨...⟩.
6 מקל מכי ובלע׳ דליום אינדיאני: קר יבש מאמץ המעים.

---

7 יוסיף בשכבת הזרע ותאות המשגל: يزيد في الباه O || ויפתח הסתומים: om. O

1 משכטראמשיר ... הנדות: om. O 2 על: om. א 4 בדליום: emend. ed. בלדיום א || וטוב לטחורים: om. א 5 מאהזהרה: om. א || ובל״ח: emend. ed. ובל״ע א || ⟨ ... ⟩: حار مسهل جيّد للنقرس ووجع الورك والظهر O

7 Fruit of the ash tree (*Fraxinus excelsior*); Rom. LNG'ʾWYŠ; Rabb. Hebr. LŠWN ṢPWR: It increases the sperm and the sexual lust; it opens obstructions and is beneficial for palpitations of the heart (heart burn).

Mem

1 Dittany (*Origanum dictamnus*): It is hot; it stimulates the flow of urine and menstrual blood (it is effective as a diuretic and emmenagogue).
2 Wild aneth (*Meum athamanticum Jacq.*); Rom. MWW: It is hot [and] good for difficult urination when it is ingested or applied as a poultice to the pubes.
3 Mastic (resin of *Pistacia lentiscus*); Rom. MŠTYQ: It is hot; it strengthens the stomach and the liver.
4 Bdellium (resin from *Balsomodendron mukul*); Rom. BDLYWM GYMYNYS: It disperses hard tumors and is good for hemorrhoids.
5 Mʾ HZHRH (= *māhīzahra*); Rom. Pʾ YRY ʾYNNS PYL; Rabb. Hebr. ʾBṬRM HBN: [It is hot and has a purgative effect; it is good for podagra and pain in the hips and back].
6 Bdellium of Mecca; Rom. DLYWM ʾYNDYʾNY: It is cold [and] dry [and] constipates the bowels.

7 "Fruit of the ash tree" (LSʾN ʾLʿṢʾPYR): Cf. IĞ 505; SHS 1:286 (Lamed 2). || "palpitations of the heart (heart burn)": Cf. Dalet 1.

1 "Dittany" (MŠKṬRʾMŠYR): Cf. IĞ 225; "Dittany … diuretic": Om. O. 2 "Wild aneth" (MW): Cf. IĞ 561. || "pubes" (הזקן התחתון): Cf. MN 1:90. 3 "Mastic" (MṢṬKY): Cf. IĞ 562; SHS 1:336 (Nun 2). 4 "Bdellium" (MQL ʾLYHWDY): Cf. IĞ 521: مقل اليهود هو الأزرق منه (*Muql al-Yahūd* ["bdellium of the Jews"] is the blue variety [*azraq*] of it). || "and is good for hemorrhoids": Om. א. 5 "Mʾ HZHRH" (= *māhīzahra*): This is a Persian term; cf. VL 2:1130 f.: "n.c. cortex radicis plantae valde niger, iecori piscis similis et pisces necans"; SC 1147: "A poisonous yellow-flowering milk-grass which, thrown into water, intoxicates the fish and brings them to the surface." Its Arabic equivalent is *māhīzahrağ* and refers to the seed of *Anamirta cocculus Wight et Arnott* (Menispermaceae); cf. SP 697; ID 2:15; SHS 1:104–105 (Alef 18). || "[It is hot and has a purgative effect; it is good for podagra and pain in the hips and back]": Transl. after O. 6 "Bdellium of Mecca" (MQL MKY): Cf. Mem 4 above.

7 מומיא ובלע׳ מומיא: טוב לרקיקת הדם וימהר חבוש שאר האברים ויועיל ממיחוש הראש הבא מצד הקור כשינתן ממנו עם שמן זנבק בנחירים.

8 מאהודאנה ובלע׳ קטפוסיא מנור או קאקמיא והוא חב אלמלך: חם ישלשל ויקיא בחזקה ויועיל מן הפדגרא.

9 מרקשיתא: חם יבש יחזק העין עם לטישה חזקה.

10 מאמיראן ובלעז סילידוניאה מנור: חם טוב ללובן העין ויחדד הראות.

11 מגאת: טוב כשיוטח על האברים הנמחצים.

12 מאזריון ובלעז לוריולה: טוב ישלשל המים בחזקה ויזיק בכבד.

13 מר ובלעז מירא ובל״ח מר: חם טוב לשעול הישן ויזכך הקול ויגרום חוג ויתן לו שינה ויהדוף הווסת ויועיל מעקיצת העקרב כשישתה.

14 מיובזג ובלע׳ אישטאפיזקרא או קפאפורגא והוא חב ⟨א⟩ל ראס והוא צמוקי ההר: חם שורף הכינים וינתק הגרב ואם ישתה ממנו מעט מזער יעורר הקיא וריבויו אפשר שימית.

---

7 טוב ... בנחירים: جيّد لنفث الدم ويسكن وجع الحلق والكسر والوثء والرضّ والفسخ وأمّا ما قيل فيه إنّه يجبر العظام جبرا تامّا فباطل بل يسرع جبار الكسر نافع من الصداع البارد إذا سعط به مع دهن زنبق O || זנבק: זנבאק א 8 בחזקה: om. O 9 מרקשיתא: מרקשיודא א 10 חם: חד ישלשל המים בחזקה add. א 11 הנמחצים: الواهنة O 12 מאזריון: emend. ed. מאזרין א ⟨ ... ⟩ ב || טוב: حارّ حديد O 13 הישן: emend. ed. הישובי א || ויהדוף: ويدرّ O

7 Mummy; Rom. MWMY’: It is good for hemoptysis [and] quickens the setting of all limbs; it is beneficial for headache caused by cold when it is applied as an errhine together with jasmine oil (extracted from *Jasminum officinale* or from *Jasminum Sambac Aitch.*).

8 Spurge (*Euphorbia Lathyris*); Rom. QṬPWSY’ MNWR or Q’QMY’; i.e., ḤB ’LMLK: It is hot; it purges and induces severe vomiting and is beneficial for podagra.

9 Marcasite: It is hot [and] dry; it strengthens the eyes and cleanses them forcefully.

10 Greater celandine (*Chelidonium maius* and Var.); Rom. SYLYDWNY’H MNWR: It is hot [and] good for leucoma, and it sharpens vision.

11 Moghat (root of *Clossostemon Bruguieri* D.C.): It is good when it is rubbed on bruised (wounded) limbs.

12 Mezereon; Rom. LWRYWLH: It is hot and sharp; it purges the [bodily] humors with force and is harmful for the liver.

13 Myrrh (resin made from *Commiphora myrrha*); Rom. MYR’; Rabb. Hebr. MR: It is hot [and] good for chronic cough; it purifies the voice, causes dizziness (stupefaction), induces sleep, stimulates the menstrual flow, and is beneficial for scorpion stings when ingested.

14 Stavesacre (*Delphinium staphisagria*); Rom. ’YŠṬ’PYZQR’ or QP’PWRG’; i.e., ḤB ’LR’S; i.e., ṢMWQY HHR: It is hot; it burns lice and eliminates mange. If a small amount is ingested, it induces vomiting; a large dosis of it can be fatal.

---

7 “Mummy” (MWMY’): Cf. M 234. ‖ “It … oil”: “It is good for hemoptysis, alleviates the pain of a sore throat and of fractures, bruises, contusions and disruptures. As for what is said that it is perfect for setting [broken] bones, that is false, [for] it [merely] accelerates the healing of fractures. It is beneficial for headache caused by cold if it is used as an errhine with jasmine oil” O. 8 “Spurge” (M’HWD’NH): Cf. IĞ 560. ‖ “ḤB ’LMLK” (*ḥabb al-mulūk*): Cf. IB 1:574. 9 “Marcasite” (MRQŠYT’): Cf. KM 2:992–997. ‖ “cleanses” (לטישה) (= Arab. جلاء): Cf. NM 4; s.v. לטישה (forthcoming). 10 “Greater celandine” (M’MYR’N): Cf. IĞ 128; DT 2:162. ‖ “hot”: “[and] sharp; it purges the water(?) forcefully” add. א. 11 “Moghat” (MG’T): This identification is the result of modern research, undertaken by Schweinfurth. In medieval Arabic medical literature, the term is erroneously used for the rind of the root of the wild pomegranate tree; cf. DT 1:82, n. 2; M 219. For the term *moghat*, cf. El S. Amin, Olfat Awad, M. Abd El Samad, and M.N. Iskander, “Isolation of estrone from moghat roots and from pollen grains of Egyptian date palm,” *Phytochemistry* 8, no. 1 (1969):295–297. ‖ “bruised (wounded) limbs”: “weak limbs” O. 12 “Mezereon (M’ZRYWN); Rom. LWRYWLH”: Cf. IĞ 391; SHS 1:103 (Alef 16). ‖ “It is hot and sharp”: Translated after O; “It is good” א. 13 “Myrrh” (MR): Cf. SHS 1:307 (Mem 8). ‖ “dizziness (stupefaction)” (חוג): Cf. NM 1:12. 14 “Stavesacre” (MYWBZG): Cf. IĞ 332; IT, Alef 33; DT 4:141.

15 מרדסנג ובלע׳ ליטרג וב״ח מרתכא: קר יועיל מן העיצום ומן הזיעה ויצמיח הבשר ויכנס ברטיות.

16 מדאד וב״מ דיו: הטיחה בו טובה לשרפת האש.

17 מראיר וב״מ מררות: כלם חמים לוטשים חשכת העין ומונעים ירידת המים בהם ומעמידים אשר ירדו בהם כדי שלא יוסיפו.

18 מגנאטיס ובלעז פירא קרמיטא: קר יבש מסגולתו שהוא יועיל למי שיתעכבו בבטנו סיגי ברזל.

אות הנון

1 נארמשך: חם יבש מחמם האצטומכה והכבד הקרים ואמרו שהוא אילן הובא מהודו יש לו רמונים קטנים פותחים כמו הורדים.

2 נטרון בלעז שלניטרי וב״מ בורית: חם לוטש מנקה האצטומכה.

3 ניל: חם קובץ מצמק המורסות התפוחות.

4 נשאדר ובלע׳ שלמוניאק: חם יועיל לנפילת ערלת הגרון והחניקה ולובן העין.

5 נאנכה וב״ל אמאוש: חם יבש מחמם האצטומכה והכבד ומגיר השתן.

---

15 העיצום: السحج O || הזיעה: نتن العرق O   16 מדאד ... האש: om. O   17 לוטשים: تجلو O || ומונעים ... יוסיפו: om. O || כדי שלא יוסיפו: ב om.   18 מגנאטיס: מאגדאטיס א מגנאטיס ... ברזל om. O || יועיל: א om.

1 נארמשך: נאבמשך א || מחמם האצטומכה והכבד הקרים: ב om. || ואמרו ... הורדים: om. O إسحاق ابن عمران: ... وهو رمانة صغيرة مفتحة كأنها وردة IB 2:471   3 התפוחות: emend. ed. הפותחות א הפתוחות ב الرهلة O   4 חם: א om.   5 נאנכה: نانخواه O

15 Silver dross; Rom. LYṬRG; Aram. MRTK': It is cold, it is beneficial for intestinal illness (dysentery) and for sweat; it regenerates flesh and should be used as a salve.

16 Ink; Rabb. Hebr. DYW: It is good for burns when it is rubbed [on the spot].

17 Bile; Rabb. Hebr. MRRWT: All [kinds of bile] are hot; they cure dimsightedness and prevent a cataract, and [once a cataract occurs] they stop it from getting worse.

18 Magnetite (lodestone, magnetic iron ore, Fe_3O_4); Rom. PYR' QRMYṬ': It is cold [and] dry; it has the specific property to be beneficial for someone if iron dross is detained in his stomach.

Nun

1 Indian rose chestnut (*Mesua ferrea*): It is hot [and] dry; it heats the cold stomach and liver; it is said that it is a tree that has been imported from India and that has small pomegranates that open like roses.

2 Natron; Rom. ŠLNYṬRY; Rabb. Hebr. BWRYT: It is hot [and] it cleanses and purifies the stomach.

3 Indigo (*Indigofera tinctoria*): It is hot [and] astringent [and] shrinks flabby tumors.

4 Sal ammoniac; Rom. ŠLMWNY'Q: It is hot [and] beneficial for a prolapsed uvula, quinsy (angina), and leucoma.

5 Bisnaga (*Ammi visnaga*); Rom. 'M'WŠ: It is hot [and] dry; it warms the stomach and liver and makes the urine flow.

15 "Silver dross" (MRDSNG): Cf. SHS 1:305 (Mem 6). ‖ "intestinal illness (dysentery)" (עיצום): Cf. Bet 13 above. ‖ "sweat": "bad smelling sweat" O. 16 "Ink" (MD'D): Cf. D 2:573–574; "Ink … the spot": Om. O. 17 "Bile" (MR'YR) (*al-mirārāt* O): Cf. D 2:576–577. ‖ "cure" (לטש) (Arab. تجلو; lit., "cleanse"): Cf. NM 4, s.v. לטש (forthcoming). ‖ "and … worse": Om. O. 18 "Magnetite" (MGN'ṬYS): Cf. SHS 1:107–108 (Alef 20): "Magnetite … stomach": Om. O.

1 "Indian rose chestnut" (N'RMŠK): Cf. IĞ 608. ‖ "it is said that it is a tree that has been imported from India and that has small pomegranates that open like roses": Cf. Isḥāq ibn 'Imrān, as quoted by Ibn al-Bayṭār (IB 2:471): "Its flower is like a small pomegranate that opens like a rose." 2 "Natron": Cf. KM 2:1082–1087; SHS 1:133 (Bet 5). ‖ "cleanses" (לוטש): Cf. Mem 17 above. 3 "Indigo" (NYL): Cf. IĞ 297, 382, 418. 4 "Sal ammoniac" (NŠ'DR): Cf. KM 2:1100–1105; IT, Shin 2. ‖ "quinsy (angina)" (חניקה, Arab. خوانيق): Cf. NM 1:94. 5 "Bisnaga" (N'NKH): Cf. IĞ 1057; SHS 1:337 (Nun 3).

6 נשאסתג ובלע׳ אמידום: קר יבש ומסגולתו התועלת מרקיקת הדם והשלשול המררי ושחין המעים וחריפות השתן וכל שכן כשיבושל בעדשים ויש שנותנים אותו בכחולים להגרת הדם המתלהבת אל העין והלחות אשר תקרה בה.

7 נפט וכן שמו ב״ח ובלעז פוג גרדישג: חם טוב לרנפלי והרוחות וכשינתן ממנו בפי הטבעת יהרוג התולעים הקטנים ויועיל מדפיקת הלב.

אות הסמך

1 סורנגאן ובלעז ארמודינטילי: חם טוב לפודגרא מוסיף בשכבת הזרע.

2 סקנקור יש אומרים שהוא הכח ובלע׳ פיש דשייט וב״מ דג ציטן: חם מעורר תאות המשגל ובסגולה כשיאכלו כליותיו.

3 סוס ובלעז ריקליציאה וב״ח שוש: טוב לגרון והריאה מוציאה מה שיש בה ומפסיק הצמא ומסיר חריפות השתן.

4 ססאליוס ובלעז שיזליוס: חם טוב לרנפלי וקשי השתן והנפח בבטן ויקל הלידה.

5 סכבינג ובלעז מאפיר: חם טוב לרוחות העבות וההדרקון והפלג וילטוש חשיכות הראות ויועיל מעקיצת העקרבים.

6 סמאק ובלעז סומאקו וב״מ אוג: קר יבש מאמץ המעים ומעבד האצטומכה.

---

6 נשאסתג ... בה: om. O   7 פוג גרדישג: פואג גראשק ב ‖ ויועיל מדפיקת הלב: om. O

1 ארמודינטיל: ארמודקטיל א ‖ חם: om. O   2 פיש: emend. ed. פוש א ‖ וב״מ: emend. ed. ומ א
3 ומסיר: om. א   5 מאפיר: שרפי ב ‖ וההדרקון: والقولنج O والصرع add. O   6 סמאק: סמאך ב ‖ אוג: emend. ed. זוג א ‖ ומעבד: دابغ O

6 Starch; Rom. ʾMYDWM: It is cold [and] dry; it has the specific property to be beneficial for hemoptysis, bilious diarrhea, intestinal ulcers, and sharp urine, especially when it is boiled with lentils. It is also put into collyria when hot blood streams to the eye and when it is affected by humors.

7 Naphtha (petroleum); it has the same name in Rabb. Hebr.; Rom. PWG GRDYŠG: It is hot [and] beneficial for asthma and winds, and when it is applied as a rectal suppository it kills small worms; it is also beneficial for palpitations of the heart (heart burn).

Samekh

1 Autumn crocus (*Colchicum autumnale*); Rom. ʾRMWDQṬYL: It is hot, good for podagra, [and] it increases the sperm.

2 Skink (*Scincus officinalis*); some say that it is HKḤ; Rom. PYŠ DŠYYṬ; Rabb. Hebr. DG ṢYṬN: It is hot; it arouses the sexual lust, especially when one eats its kidneys.

3 Licorice (Glycyrrhiza glabra); Rom. RYQLYṢYʾH; Rabb. Hebr. ŠWŠ: It is good for the throat and lungs; it expels the [superfluities] that are retained in them and lessens the thirst and neutralizes the sharpness of the urine.

4 Massilian hartwort (*Seseli tortuosum*); Rom. ŠYZLYWS: It is hot [and] good for asthma, difficult urination, flatulence in the stomach, and it eases childbirth.

5 Sagapenum (i.e., gum resin of the Persian giant fennel [*Ferula persica*, olim: *Ferula szowitziana*]); Rom. Mʾ PYR: It is hot [and] good for thick winds, colic, and hemiplegia; it cures dimsightedness and is beneficial for scorpion stings.

6 Sumac (*Rhus coriaria*); Rom. SWMʾQW; Rabb. Hebr. ʾWG: It is cold [and] dry; it constipates the bowels and strengthens the stomach.

---

6 "Starch" (NŠʾSTG): Cf. IĞ 498; SHS 1:217 (Ḥet 14); "Starch ... humors": Om. O. 7 "Naphtha (petroleum)" (NPṬ): Cf. KM 2:1087–1089. || "palpitations of the heart (heart burn)": Cf. Dalet 1 above.

1 "Autumn crocus" (SWRNGʾN): Cf. IĞ 654. || "It is hot": Om. O. 2 "Skink" (SQNQWR): Cf. SHS 1:277–278 (Kaf 25). || Hebr. DG ṢYṬN features in the anonymous translation of Maimonides, *On Coitus* 8 (ed. Gerrit Bos, forthcoming), as DG ṢYYṬ for Arab. *saqanqūr* ("skink"). || According to Dietrich (DT 2:53), the parts around the kidneys, dried and consumed with wine, were used to increase sexual vigour. 3 "Licorice" (SWS): Cf. IĞ 695; SHS 1:522–523 (Shin 51). 4 "Massilian hartwort" (SSʾLYWS): Cf. IĞ 420. 5 "Sagapenum" (SKBYNG): Cf. IĞ 653. || "colic": Cf. Bet 6 above. || "cures dimsightedness": Cf. Mem 17 above. 6 "Sumac" (SMʾQ): Cf. IĞ 1003; SHS 1:93–94 (Alef 3). || "strengthens" (מעבד): Cf. Alef 22 above.

7 סקמוניא ובלעז אשקמוניאה: משלשלת המרה הכרכומית בחזקה ומזקת האצטומכה והמעים והכבד ואם ילקח ממנו יותר מן הראוי תמית.

8 סנא ובלעז שינא שאנה וב״ח סינים או סנה: ישלשל החלטים הנשרפים מן הגרב והחכוך.

9 שאדוראן(?) ויש מן המפרשים ⟨...⟩ לפיש אמאטיטוש: קר קובץ עוצר הדם ומונע נשירת השער.

10 סקולופנדריון: חם ישלשל טוב לטחול העב והטפת השתן.

11 סבסתאן ובלעז שבשתאן: שוה החמימות מרכך הגרון והחזה.

12 סנדרוס ובלעז קלאשא: יועיל לרקיקת הדם והטחורים.

13 סרו ובלעז סאפיריסוס: עליו ואגוזיו חמים קובצים ⟨טובים⟩ לפיתקא כשיחובש בו.

14 סעד ובלעז סיפרום אורטירגאנגלי וב״ח סיגלי: חם יבש מחמם האצטומכה והכבד ומפרך החצץ טוב לקיטור והעיפוש בפה או באף.

---

7 ומזקת: ומחזק ב || ואם ילקח ממנו יותר מן הראוי תמית: om. O 8 סנא ... והחכוך: om. O 9 קובץ: כובש א 10 סקולופנדריון: emend. ed. סקואלופנדרין א סקולופדריון ב 11 שוה החמימות: om. O

7 Scammony (*Convolvulus scammonia*); Rom. ʾŠQMWNYʾH: It purges the yellow bile with [a strong purgative power]; it is harmful for the stomach, intestines, and liver, and if one takes more than appropriate, it is fatal.

8 Senna (and its numerous species, such as *Senna alexandrina Mill.* [= *Cassia angustifolia*] or *Senna italica Mill.* [= *Cassia obovata*]); Rom. ŠYNʾ, ŠʾNʾ; Rabb. Hebr. SYNYM or SNH: It purges the burned humors caused by mange and itch.

9 ŠʾDWRʾN; some commentators [say that it is identical with] haematite (= Arab. ŠʾḎNH): It is cold [and] astringent; it stops bleedings and prevents loss of hair (alopecia).

10 Hart's tongue (*Scolopendrium vulgare*, or *Asplenium scolopendrium*): It is hot [and] has a purgative effect, [and] is good for a thick, enlarged spleen and for strangury.

11 Sebesten (i.e., the fruit of the sebesten tree [*Cordia Myxa*]); Rom. ŠBŠTʾN: It is moderate in heat; it softens the throat and the chest.

12 Resin from the sandarac tree (*Callitris quadrivalvis*); Rom. QLʾŠʾ: It is beneficial for hemoptysis and hemorrhoids.

13 Cypress (*Cupressus sempervivens* and Var.); Rom. SʾPYRYSWS: Its leaves and nuts are hot [and] astringent [and] good for hernia when they are applied to it as a poultice.

14 Galingale (*Cyperus longus* and Var.); Rom. SYPRYM ʾWRṬYRGʾNGLY; Rabb. Hebr. SYGLY: It is hot [and] dry; it heats the stomach and liver and pulverizes [intestinal] stones; it is good for bad breath and putridity in the mouth or nose.

---

7 "Scammony" (SQMWNYʾ): Cf. IT, Alef 34. 8 "Senna" (SNʾ): Cf. SHS 1:372 (Samekh 39); "Senna … itch": Om. O. 9 "ŠʾDWRʾN": I.e., *sādarwān* (سادروان); cf. DT 1:39, n. 5: "a black odourless juice from the roots of different kinds of terebinth and other trees" (trans. ed.). ‖ "some commentators [say that it is identical with] haematite": Cf. IBF 1152: "We find the term (i.e., ŠʾDWRʾN) in a note in Ms 1071 in the Persian form شیاه داوران … But the true meaning of this word, according to Persian dictionaries, is 'pearls or glass jewelry worn as an ornament by rich persons'" (trans. ed.). 10 "Hart's tongue" (SQWLWPNDRYWN): The term can also refer to the "rusty-back fern" (*Ceterach officinarum*, or *Asplenium ceterach*); cf. IĞ 641. ‖ "strangury" (הטפת השתן; Arab. تقتير البول): Cf. NM 3:64. 11 "Sebesten" (SBSTʾN): Cf. IĞ 666; SHS 1:148 (Gimel 3). ‖ "It is moderate in heat": Om O. 12 "Resin from the sandarac tree" (SNDRWS): Cf. IT, Qof 5. 13 "Cypress" (SRW): Cf. IĞ 235; IT, Nun 1. ‖ "hernia" (פיתקא): Cf. SHS 1:428 (Pe 48). 14 "Galingale" (SʿD): Cf. IĞ 651; SHS 1:374–375 (Samekh 44). ‖ "bad breath" (קיטור, Arab. بخر): Cf. NM 2:18, and correction NM 3:268.

15 סרטאן ובלעז קרנק וב״ח סרטן: מי הבשר יועיל למי שיש לו שחפת ויוסיף בשכבת הזרע. והסרטן ההודיי קר יבש יועיל ללחות העין כשיוכחל בו והסרטאן הנהרי כששורפין אותו ומערבין דשנו עם הגנטיאנה וישתה ממנו בכל יום משקל זהוב בתירוש מבושל יועיל מנשיכת הכלב השוטה ואם יבושל חי בחלב יועיל מעקיצת הרמשים והעקרבים ובשרו יועיל עוד לשחפת ויוסיף בשכבת הזרע.

16 סנבל ובלעז אשפיק וב״מ שבולת: חם טוב לאצטומכה ולכבד הקרים ויגיר השתן.

17 סליכה ובלעז קשיאה ליניא וב״ח קלפה: חמה מחדדת הראות ומגרת השתן.

18 סאדג ובלעז מלאבטרום: יועיל מדפיקת הלב והאד.

19 שד: חם טוב לכאב העצבים והרוחות.

אות העין

1 עצה אלראעי ובלעז וירגא פשטורא וב״מ מקל הרועה וב״ח חוטרא רעיא: קר טוב למורסות החמות ולהבת האצטומכה כשיחובש בו.

2 עאקר קרחה ובלעז פליטרי וב״מ הרזפא: חם יבש טוב לכאב השנים ושחין הפה.

---

15 מי הבשר: ⟨מ⟩ימי בשרו ב لحمه O ‖ והסרטן ... הזרע: om. O 17 חמה: يابسة add. O 18 יועיל: حارّ يدرّ البول وينفع O

1 עצה אלראעי: emend. ed. אלרע א ב om. 2 פליטרי: emend. ed. פלנטרי א פליטררי ב ‖ חם יבש: om. א ‖ יבש: om. O

15 Crab; Rom. QRNQ; Rabb. Hebr. SRṬN: The bouillon of its flesh is beneficial for someone who suffers from phthisis and increases the sperm. Indian crab is cold [and] dry and beneficial for humors in the eye when it is applied as a collyrium. If one burns river crab and mixes its ashes with gentian (*Gentiana lutea*) and drinks every day a dosis of one ZHWB (lit., gold coin) with boiled grape juice, it is beneficial for mad dog bites, and if it is boiled while it is still alive with milk, it is beneficial for stings or bites of vermin and scorpions; its flesh is also beneficial for phthisis and it increases the sperm.

16 Spikenard (*Nardostachys jatamansi*); Rom. ʾŠPYQ; Rabb. Hebr. ŠBWLT: It is hot [and] good for a cold stomach and liver; it makes the urine flow.

17 Cassia (*Cinnamomum cassia*); Rom. QŠYʾ H LYNYʾ; Rabb. Hebr. QLPH: It is hot; it sharpens vision and makes the urine flow.

18 SʾDG; Rom. MLʾBṬRWM: It is beneficial for palpitations of the heart (heart burn) and [bad] breath.

19 SK: It is hot and good for painful nerves (neuralgia) and winds.

Ayin

1 Knotgrass (*Polygonum aviculare*); Rom. WYRGʾ PŠṬWRʾ, Rabb. Hebr. MQL HRWʿH; Aram. ḤWṬʿ RʿYʾ: It is hot and good for inflamed tumors and inflammation of the stomach when it is applied as a poultice to them.

2 Pellitory (*Anacyclus pyrethrum*); Rom. PLYṬRY; Rabb. Hebr. HRZPʾ: It is hot [and] dry [and] good for toothache and pustules in the mouth.

---

15 "Crab" (SRṬʾN): Cf. SHS 1:429 (Ṣade 1). || "The bouillon of its flesh": "its flesh" O. || "Indian … sperm": Om. O. || "ZHWB (lit., gold coin)": The term stands for Arab. مثقال (i.e., 4.46 grams); cf. NM 4, s.v. זהוב (forthcoming). 16 "Spikenard" (SNBL): Cf. IǦ 600; SHS 1: 501–502 (Shin 10). 17 "Cassia" (SLYKH): Cf. SHS 1:466 (Qof 34). || "hot": "dry" add. O. 18 "SʾDG": Arab. *sādaǧ* is possibly *Laurus malabathrum*, or *Laurus cassia*, folia indica; cf. SP 361; DT 1:9. || "It is beneficial": "It is hot, it makes the urine flow and is beneficial" O. || "palpitations of the heart (heart burn)": Cf. Dalet 1 above. 19 "SK" (*sukk*): A compound remedy; Isḥāq Ibn ʿImrān (following Ibn al-Bayṭār) states that there are four kinds, foremost that prepared with musk and other ingredients (cf. IB 2:32; IBF 1201; D 1:666).

1 "Knotgrass" (ʿṢH ʾLʾ ʿY): Cf. IǦ 980. || "MQL HRWʿH": Cf. NM 2:15. 2 "Pellitory" (ʿʾQR QRḤH): Cf. IǦ 1008; SHS 1:181–182 (He 2). || "dry": Om O.

3 ערוק צפרי הוא שני מינים קטון וגדול הקטון שמו מאמירן שהיא בלעז סילידוניה פיקה וזה שמו סילידוניה גראנ⟨ד⟩א: חם לוטש יחדד הראות ויסיר הלובן מן העין.

4 ענב אלתעלב ובלעז מברילה וב״מ ענב השועל: קר טוב לכבד המתלהבת.

5 ענאב: חם בשווי מרכך הגרון ומזכך הדם מזהים מתעכב הירידה מהאצטומכה.

6 ערער ובלע׳ גנברי: טוב יחמם ויגיר השתן ודם הנדות ויועיל לאצטומ׳.

7 עלך אלאנבאט חם טוב לסדקים והשחין ובלעז טרבנטינא.

8 עצפר ובלעז שפראן אורטואל וב״מ חריע: חם טוב לבהק ולנתק.

9 עליק ובלעז רומזי וב״מ קמשונים: מימיו חמים והזורק אותם על הפרעושים יהרגם והוא שורף השער.

10 עוסג ובלעז ארנש וב״מ אטד: קר יבש ישקיט המורסות כשינתן עליהם.

אות הפא

1 פלפל ובלעז פברי וב״ח פלפל: חם טוב לכאב העצבים.

---

5 ומזכך: يطفئ O ‖ מזהים: מזהיר א وخم O 6 טוב: om. ב حبّه O ‖ ויגיר השתן ודם הנדות: om. O 7 עלך אלאנבאט: עלג אלנבאט א ‖ והשחין: والبثور والقروح في الفم O ‖ טרבנטינא: וב״ח חריע add. א 8 חריע: emend. ed. אריע א ‖ חם: om. א ‖ נתק: كلف O 9 עליק ... השער: om. O

10 עוסג: om. א עוסג ... עליהם: om. O ‖ קר יבש ישקיט המורסות כשינתן עליהם: om. א

1 פלפל ... העצבים: om. O

3 "Yellow roots" (ʿRWQ ṢFRY): It consists of two kinds: small and large; the small [kind] is called M'MYRN (i.e., celandine, *Chelidonium majus*!), that is Rom. SYLYDWNYH PYQH, and the [other, large kind is called] SYLYDWNYH GR'N[D]' (i.e., curcuma, *Curcuma longa*). It is hot, it has a cleansing effect, sharpens the vision, and cures leucoma.

4 Black nightshade (*Solanum nigrum*); Rom. MBRYLH; Rabb. Hebr. ʿNB HŠWʿL: It is cold [and] good for an inflamed liver.

5 Jujube (*Zizyphus jujuba*): It is moderately hot; it softens the throat [and] purifies the blood; it is heavy [on the stomach], hard to digest, [and] slow to be digested.

6 Common juniper (Juniperus communis); Rom. GNBRY: Its berries have a heating effect; they make the urine and the menstrual blood flow and are beneficial for the stomach.

7 Mastic (the resin of *Pistacia lentiscus*): It is hot [and] good for cracks and pustules. In Romance [it is called] ṬRBNṬYN'.

8 Safflower (*Carthamus tinctorius*); Rom. ŠPR'N 'RṬW'L; Rabb. Hebr. ḤRYʿ: It is hot and good for *bahaq* and freckles.

9 Blackberry (*Rubus fruticosus*); Rom. RWMZY; Rabb. Hebr. QMŠWNYM: Its juice is hot; it kills fleas if one pours it on them and it burns the hair.

10 Boxthorn (*Lycium sp.*); Rom. 'RNŠ; Rabb. Hebr. 'ṬD: It is cold [and] dry; it alleviates [the pain of] tumors when it is put on them.

Pe

1 Pepper (*Piper nigrum*); Rom. PBRY; Rabb. Hebr. PLPL: It is hot [and] good for painful nerves (neuralgia).

---

3 "M'MYRN" (*māmīrān*): Cf. IĞ 1040; DT 2:162; M 205, 241. || "has a cleansing effect" (לוטש): Cf. Mem 17 above. 4 "Black nightshade" (ʿNB 'LTʿLB): Cf. IĞ 459; SHS 1: 379–380 (Ayin 4). 5 "Jujube" (ʿN'B): Cf. IĞ 736. || "purifies the blood": "extinguishes [the heat of] the blood" O. || "hard to digest" (מזהים): Translated after the Arabic وخم. 6 "Common juniper" (ʿRʿR): Cf. IĞ 27; SHS 1:100 (Alef 12). || "berries": Translated after O; א has "[it is] good." 7 "Mastic" (ʿLK 'L-'NB'Ṭ) (lit., "gum of the Nabataeans"): Cf. IĞ 83; SHS 1:299 (Lamed 29). || "pustules": "pustules and ulcers in the mouth" O. 8 "Safflower" (ʿṢPR): Cf. IĞ 66; SHS 1:209 (Ḥet 1). || Cf. Zayin 2 above. || "freckles": Cf. Bet 10 above. 9 "Blackberry" (ʿLYQ): Cf. IĞ 731; SHS 1:467 (Qof 35); "Blackberry ... the hair": Om O. 10 "Boxthorn" (ʿWS'G): Cf. IĞ 61; SHS 1:124 (Alef 44); "Boxthorn ... them": Om O.

1 "Pepper" (PLPL): Cf. DT 2:43; "Pepper ... (neuralgia)": Om. O.

2 פו ⟨ובלעז⟩ ולריאנה: חם דק מפרד החצץ ומגיר השתן.

3 פרביון ובלע׳ איפורבי: חם מאד ישלשל המים ויועיל מן ההדרקון והפלג.

4 פילזהרג הוא לשון פרס וב״מ מררת הפיל ובלעז ליסיאום: יחזק השער כשינתן על הראש.

5 פראסיון ובלעז פראשיום וב״מ לפסן: חם טוב לרנפלי וקושי הנישום והירקון.

6 פאוניא ובלעז פאווינה: טוב לפחד הנערים כשתולין אותו עליהם ו⟨כש⟩מקטירין בו האף יועיל מן הכפיון.

7 פלפמוניאה: חמה טובה להדרקון והרוחות ותשלשל המים בכח מועילה מן הפלג והדומה לו וכשכוחלין ⟨אותה⟩ תועיל מן התחלת המים.

8 פופל ובלעז אוילאנא אינדיגא וב״מ לוז הודיי: קר טוב למורסות כשיוטח בו עליהם.

9 פנגנכסת ענינו בלשון פרס חמשה עלין ובלעז זינושקא שטוש וקראו אותו הישמעאלים אילן אברהם: חם יועיל לעובי הטחול ויסיר הקושי.

10 פוה ובלע׳ רוביה וב״ח פואה: חמה מגרת השתן ודם הנדות ותועיל מן הבהק והצרעת כשיוטח בה.

---

2 דק מפרד החצץ: om. O   3 פרביון: פרבון א ‖ מאד: om. ב ‖ המים: بقوة add. O ‖ ויועיל מן ההדרקון והפלג: نافع من الفالج ونحوه وإن أكتحل نفع من ابتداء الماء O   4 כשינתן על הראש: om. O   5 פראסיון: פראסאן א   6 עליהם: ومن الصرع add. O ‖ האף: אף החמורים א   7 פלפמוניאה: emend. ed. פלגמוניאה א פלגמוניה ב ‖ להדרקון: للقولنج O ‖ ותשלשל המים בכח מועילה מן הפלג והדומה לו וכשכוחלין ⟨אותה⟩ תועיל מן התחלת המים: om. O   8 למורסות: الحارّة add. O   9 פנגנכסת ... הקושי: om. O ‖ וקראו: emend. ed. וקראום א ⟨...⟩ ב   10 פוה: فوة الصبغ O ‖ רוביה: emend. ed. רוגיה א ⟨...⟩ ב

2 Valerian (*Valerina officinalis*?); [Rom.] WLRY'NH: It is hot [and] fine; it pulverizes [intestinal] stones and makes the urine flow.

3 Resin spurge (*Euphorbia resinera*); Rom. 'YPWRBY: It is very hot; it purges the [bodily] humors and is beneficial for a colic and hemiplegia.

4 Buckthorn (PYLZHRG); this is a Persian term; Rabb. Hebr. MRRT HPYL; Rom. LYSY'WM: It strengthens the hair when it is put on the head.

5 White horehound (*Marrubium vulgare*); Rom. PR'ŠYWM; Rabb. Hebr. LPSN: It is hot [and] good for asthma, difficulty of breathing (dyspnea), and jaundice.

6 Peony (*Paeonia officinalis*); Rom. P'WWYNH: It is good for children affected by fear if it is hung [around their neck], and it is beneficial for epilepsy if it is applied as an errhine.

7 Root of the long pepper plant (*Piper longum*): It is hot [and good] for a colic and winds; it purges the humors with force; it is beneficial for hemiplegia and the like and for a beginning [cataract] when it is used as an eye-salve.

8 Areca nut (fruit of the Areca palm [*Areca catechu*]); Rom. 'BYL'NH 'YNDYG'; Rabb. Hebr. LWZ HWDYY: It is cold [and] good for tumors when it is rubbed on them.

9 Chaste tree (*Vitex agnus castus*); in Persian it means "five leaves"; Rom. ZYNWŠQ' ŠṬWŠ; the Arabs call it "tree of Abraham": It is hot [and] beneficial for thickness of the spleen and removes [its] hardness.

10 Madder, (*Rubia tinctorum*); Rom. RWBYH; Rabb. Hebr. PW'H: It is hot; it makes the urine and the menstrual blood flow; it is beneficial for *bahaq* and leprosy when it is rubbed on them.

---

2 "Valerian" (PW): Cf. DT 1:8. ‖ "[and] fine; it pulverizes [intestinal] stones": Om. O. 3 "Resin spurge" (PRBYWN): Cf. IĞ 1009; IT, Alef 9. ‖ "humors": "with force" add. O. ‖ "and is beneficial for a colic and hemiplegia": "and is beneficial for hemiplegia and if it is applied in an eye-salve, it is beneficial for the beginning of moisture (a cataract)" O. ‖ "colic": Cf. Bet 6 above. 4 "Buckthorn" (PYLZHRG): From Persian *fīl zahra*, lit., "elephant's bile" (cf. VL 2:702), the Persian term is a synonym for *ḥuḍaḍ*; the latter term was chosen by Ḥunayn for Greek λύκιον ("buckthorn"). The modern identification of this plant is very difficult; it is possibly identical with *Rhamnus infectoria*; cf. DT 1:69. ‖ "MRRT HPYL" (מררת הפיל): Cf. NM 2:15. ‖ "when it is put on the head": Om O. 5 "White horehound" (PR'SYWM): Cf. IĞ 648; SHS 1:285 (Lamed 1). 6 "Peony" (P'WNY'): Cf. IĞ 378, 761; SHS 1:520 (Shin 46). 7 "Root of the long pepper plant" (PLPMWNY'H): Cf. IĞ 331; M 310. ‖ "colic": Cf. Bet 6 above. ‖ "it ... eye-salve": Om. O. 8 "Areca nut" (PWPL): Cf. IĞ 776; SHS 1:300 (Lamed 30). ‖ "tumors": "inflamed tumors" O. 9 "Chaste tree" (PNGNKST): Cf. IĞ 116; SHS 1:114 (Alef 30); Bet 14 above; "Chaste tree ... hardness": Om. O. 10 "Madder" (PWH): Cf. IĞ 481. ‖ "PW'H": Cf. JD 1138. ‖ Cf. Zayin 2 above.

11 פלנגה: חמה יבשה.

12 פודנג ובלעז פוליג וב״מ יועזר: חם יבש טוב לרנפלי הישן ועכוב השתן.

13 פצה וב״מ כסף: קרה טובה לדפיקת הלב.

14 פאשרה ובלע׳ בידיליה: חמה לוטשת הנתק והבהק.

15 פאשרשין: יגיר השתן ודם הנדות ויועיל מן הכפיון.

16 פאריקון ובלעז יופארקי: חם דק יפתח הסתומים ויועיל מכאב הירך.

17 פאפסיום(?): הוא סחיטת זקן התיש: קר קובץ מאמץ המעים.

אות הצדי

1 צבר ובלעז אילוואי וב״ח אילווא: חם ישלשל המרה הכרכומית וינקה הראש והאצטומ׳ ויצמיח הבשר.

2 צמג ובלעז גומא וב״ח קומוס: קר רטוב ישקיט הצמא לקרירותו ויאמץ המעים.

---

12 ועכוב: וערוב א   14 הנתק: للكلف O   15 פאשרשין: emend. ed. פאשיר שיר א פאשרש⟨...⟩ ב   16 פאריקון ... הירד: om. O

2 צמג ... המעים: om. O ‖ קומוס: החלמי א add.

11 PLNGH: It is hot [and] dry.

12 Mint (*Mentha sp.*); Rom. PWLYG; Rabb. Hebr. YW'ZR: It is hot [and] dry; it is good for chronic asthma and dysuria.

13 Silver; Rabb. Hebr. KSP: It is cold [and] good for palpitations of the heart (heart burn).

14 Bryony (possibly *Bryonia dioica* [red bryony]); Rom. BYDYLYH: It is hot and cures freckles and *bahaq*.

15 White bryony (*Bryonia alba*): It makes the urine and menstrual blood flow and it is beneficial for epilepsy.

16 Hypericum; Rom. YWP'RQY: It is hot [and] fine; it opens obstructions and is beneficial for pain in the hips.

17 P'PSYWM(?); i.e., the extract of goatsbeard (*Tragopogon porrifolius*): It is cold [and] astringent, [and] it constipates the bowels.

Ṣade

1 Aloe (*Aloe vera*); Rom. 'YLWW'Y; Rabb. Hebr. 'YLWW': It is hot; it purges the yellow bile, cleanses the head and stomach, and regenerates flesh.

2 Gum; Rom. GWM'; Rabb. Hebr. QWMWS: It is cold [and] moist; it lessens thirst because of its coldness and constipates the bowels.

---

11 "PLNGH": According to Ibn Ǧanāḥ (IǦ 317), Arab. فلنجة refers to the same plant as ZRNB (cf. Zayin 10 above and M 137): زرنب هو فلنجة من الحاوي، وفي اللغة: زرنب هو فلنجة ضرب من الطيب *Zarnab* is *falanǧa*, according to the *Ḥāwī*. From the lexicographical literature: *Zarnab* is *falanǧa*; it ranks among aromatic substances. 12 "Mint" (PWDNG): Cf. IǦ 770; SHS 1:258–259 (Yod 17). 13 "Silver" (PṢH): Cf. KM 867–870. ‖ "palpitations of the heart (heart burn)": Cf. Dalet 1 above. 14 "Bryony" (P'ŠRH): Cf. IǦ 277. ‖ "freckles": Cf. Bet 10 above. ‖ Cf. Zayin 2 above. 15 "White bryony" (*fāšarašīn*): Cf. IBF 1655; see also DT 4:175; s.v. *fāšaraštīn*. 16 "Hypericum" (P'RYQWN): For its different species, see DT 3:146; see also IǦ 274. According to DT 3:146, n. 1, the Arabic term *fārīqūn* features in secondary literature in Ibn Ǧulǧul; the regular term is *hayūfārīqūn* (cf. DT 3:146) and features in entry He 5. This entry is missing in O. 17 "P'PSYWM(?)": The term is possibly a corruption of PR'SYWN, Arab. فراسيون; Greek πράσιον; i.e., "white horehound" (*Marrubium vulgare*); cf. DT 3:99. ‖ "i.e., the extract of goatsbeard (*Tragopogon porrifolius*)": This identification is mistaken, for goatsbeard and its properties, cf. Samekh 6 above.

1 "Aloe" (ṢBR): Cf. SHS 1:110 (Alef 23); IT, Alef 13. 2 "Gum; Rom. GWM'; Rabb. Hebr. QWMWS": Cf. SHS 1:451 (Qof 7), where the Romance and Hebrew parallel terms feature for "Gum arabic" (ṢMG 'RBY).

3 צמג ערבי ובלעז גומא ארביקא וב״ח קומוס: קר יאמץ המעים ומועיל מן העיצום.

4 צדף ובלעז קוקליא וב״מ נרתיק: לוטש השינים שרוף והכותש אותו נא ויחבש בו שרפת האש יבריא אותה.

5 צוע(?): מועיל משלשול הבטן ומן השחין הנקרא אלקלאע בתכלית התועלת.

אות הקוף

1 קיסום: קר יכנס בסמי העין ויועיל מעפוש השינים וחפירתם.

2 קרדמנה ובלעז קראוי שלואיג וב״ח קרבס הרים: חמה טובה לכפיון והרנפלי והפלג ותוציא גרגרי הדלועין מן הבטן ותועיל מעקיצת עקרב.

3 קנטוריון ובלעז סינטוריא: ישלשל הליחה התפלה טוב למכאובי העצבים וההדרקון.

4 קנביל הוא עפר מתקנים בו קדרות האבנים והחרס הנשבר ונוטה אל האדמימות והוא מובא מברקא: חם יוציא גרגרי הדלועים מן הבטן.

---

4 לוטש: يجلو O

1 קיסום: emend. ed. קיסור אב قيسوم O || ויועיל מעפוש השינים וחפירתם: ويجلو الأسنان O

3 קנטוריון: קטוריון א || טוב: om. א || וההדרקון: والقولنج O   4 קנביל ... הבטן: om. ב || הוא עפר מתקנים בו קדרות האבנים החרס הנשבר ונוטה אל האדמימות והוא מובא מברקא: om. O قال غيره تربة حمراء يشوبها صفرة تشعب بها قدور البرام إذا انكسرت ويقال أنها توجد على وجه الأرض بخراسان IB 2:289

3 Gum arabic (*Acacia arabica*); Rom. GWM' 'RBYQ'; Rabb. Hebr. QWMWS: It is cold; it constipates the bowels and is beneficial for intestinal illness (dysentery).

4 Pearl oyster (sea shell); Rom. QWQLY'; Rabb. Hebr. NRTYQ: When they are burned [and applied] they clean (whiten) the teeth, and when they are raw and pulverized and then applied they cure burns.

5 ṢW'(?): It is extremely beneficial for diarrhea and for the ulceration called "qilā'" (aphthae).

Qof

1 Southernwood (*Artemisia abrotanum*): It is cold [and] used as part of eye remedies; it is beneficial for putrefaction of the teeth and for cavities.

2 Wild (bastard) cumin (*Lagoecia cuminoides*); Rom. QR'WY ŠLW'YG; Rabb. Hebr. QRBS HRYM: It is hot; it is good for epilepsy, asthma, and hemiplegia; it expels tapeworms from the stomach and is beneficial for scorpion stings.

3 Knapweed (*Centaurea centaurium*) (or common centaury [*Erythraea centaurium*]); Rom. SYNṬWRY': It purges the crude humors; it is good for painful nerves (neuralgia) and for colic.

4 Kamala; i.e., the reddish earth used for repairing broken stone and earthenware pots, and it is imported from BRQ' (*Barqā*; i.e., Cyrenaica): It is hot [and] expels tapeworms from the stomach.

---

3 "Gum arabic" (ṢMG 'RBY): Cf. SHS 1:451 (Qof 7). || "intestinal illness (dysentery)": Cf. Bet 13 and Mem 15 above. 4 "Pearl oyster (sea shell)" (ṢDP): Cf. SHS 1:341–342 (Nun 10). || "clean (whiten)" (לוטש): Cf. Mem 17. 5 "ṢW'(?): It is extremely beneficial for diarrhea and for the ulceration called 'qilā'' (aphthae)": Om. O.

1 "Southernwood" (QYSWM): Cf. IĞ 858. || "it is beneficial for putrefaction of the teeth and for caries": "it cleans the teeth" O. 2 "Wild (bastard) cumin" (QRDMNH): Cf. M 335; according to Dietrich (DT 1:5), it could be true cardamom (*Elettaria cardamomum*); see also IĞ 815; SHS 1:468 (Qof 37). || "tapeworms": Cf. Kaf 7. 3 "Knapweed" (QNṬRYWN): Cf. IĞ 857. || "colic": Cf. Bet 6 above. 4 "Kamala" (QNBYL): Cf. IĞ 823: "a red dye produced by the plant Mallotus philippensis"; "Kamala ... stomach": Om. ב. || "i.e., the reddish earth used for repairing broken stone and earthenware pots, and it is imported from BRQ'": Om. O; cf. IB 2:289 (= IBF 1842): "Someone else said that it is red earth that is mixed with yellow and that is used to repair earthernware pots when they are broken; it is said that it can be found on the surface of the earth in Khorasan" (trans. ed.). || "BRQ' (*Barqā*; i.e., Cyrenaica)": Cf. KM 1:343–344, s.v. تربة برقة (*turbat Barqa)/تربة برقا (*turbat Barqā*). || "tapeworms": Cf. Kaf 7 above.

5 קאקלא ובלעז קרדמומי: חמה מחממת האצטומכא ומשקטת האצטניסות.

6 קנה ⟨בלע׳⟩ סיטרולי או גלבנום: חם יגיר דם הנדות ויתיר הרוחות וימשמש חזירים ויצמיח הבשר.

7 קלימיה אלדהב הוא סיג הזהב תסיר לובן העין ותכנס בכחול וסיג הכסף טוב לגרב אשר בגוף ולשחין העין.

8 קרט: קר מאמץ המעים.

9 קלקנת: אוכל חם יש בו קביצות יסיר הטחורים מן האף.

10 קלקטאר: לבן ינגב שכבת הזרע ויסיר התאוה.

11 קלקדיס ואלסורי: מנגבים החבלה ופעולת אלסורי יותר גדולה.

12 קרטם ובלעז גראנא דשאפראן: חם יבש מוסיף בשכבת הזרע ומזיק אל האסטו׳.

13 קטראן: חם מועיל לגרב מגיר דם הנדות ומפיל העובר ומונע שכבת הזרע מן הזריעה.

14 קאקלי: ישלשל המים ויגיר החלב והשתן.

---

5 קאקלא: קאקלה ב ‖ האצטניסות: القيء O 6 הנדות: بقوة add. O ‖ ויצמיח הבשר: om. א 7 אלדהב: لطيف add. O ‖ ותכנס בכחול: om. O 8 קרט: emend. ed. קרץ אב قرط O ובלעז קלאשא והוא אלסנדרוס add. א ‖ המעים: add. א 9 קלקנת ... האף: om. א 10 קלקטאר ... התאוה: om. א 11 קלקדיס ... גדולה: om. O ‖ ואלסורי: והוא מין ממיני הקלקנתוס add. א ‖ החבלה: emend. ed. הבהלה א הבלה ב 12 קרטם ובלעז גראנא דשאפראן: om. ב ‖ חם ... האסטו׳: חם מועיל לגרב מגיר דם הנדות ומפיל העובר ומונע שכבת הזרע מן הזריעה א ‖ יבש: يلين البطن O 13 קטראן ... מן הזריעה: om. א ‖ חם: جدّا add. O 14 המים: המעים א

5 Black cardamom (*Amomum subulatum*) (or common cardamom [*Elettaria cardamomum*]); Rom. QRDMWMY: It is hot; it heats the stomach and relieves nausea.

6 Galbanum (gum resin of *Ferula galbaniflua*); Rom. SYṬRWLY or GLBNWM: It is hot; it makes the menstrual blood flow, dissolves winds and mumps, and regenerates flesh.

7 Gold cadmia; i.e., scoria of gold: It cures leucoma and is [beneficial when it is used] as part of an eye-salve. Scoria of silver is good for mange affecting the body and for ulcers in the eye.

8 Egyptian clover (*Trifolium alexandrinum*): It is cold [and] constipates the bowels.

9 QLQNT (a type of vitriol): It is corroding, astringent, and removes nasal polyps.

10 QLQṬ'R (a type of vitriol): It is white; it dries the sperm and takes the sexual lust away.

11 QLQDYS (a type of vitriol) and 'LSWRY (a type of vitriol): They dry wounds(?), but the effect of 'LSWRY is stronger.

12 Safflower (*Carthamus tinctorius*) seed; Rom. GR'N' DŠ'PR'N: It is hot [and] dry; it increases the sperm and is bad for the stomach.

13 Tar (or liquid pitch): It is hot; it is good for mange; it makes the menstrual blood flow; it causes a miscarriage and prevents the sperm from being fertile.

14 Saltwort (*Salsola kali, S. soda, Suaeda vera Forssk.*): It purges the humors and makes the mothermilk and urine flow.

---

5 "Black cardamom" (Q'QL'): Cf. IĞ 280. ‖ "nausea": Cf. Bet 10 above. 6 "Galbanum" (QNH): Cf. IĞ 151. ‖ "flow": "with force" add. O. ‖ "and regenerates flesh": Om. א. 7 "Gold cadmia" (QLYMYH 'LDHB): Cf. KM 1:269–271. ‖ "It cures": "It is fine (refining) [and] cures" O. ‖ "and is [beneficial when it is used] as part of an eye-salve": Om. O. 8 "Egyptian clover" (QRṬ): Cf. IĞ 883. 9 "QLQNT" (*qalqant*): I.e., a type of vitriol: according to Meyerhof (M 140), *qalqant*, *qaldadīs* (see Qof 11), and *qulquṭār* (see Qof 10) are all of them impure vitriols, above all iron sulfates; see also KM 601–615; "QLQNT ... polyps": Om. א. ‖ "polyps" (טחורים): Cf. NM 2:12. 10 "QLQṬ'R" (*qulquṭār*): Cf. entry QLQNT; "QLQṬ ... away": Om. אO. 11 "QLQDYS" (*qalqadīs*): Cf. entry QLQNT; "QLQDYS ... stronger": Om. O. ‖ "'LSWRY" (*al-sūrī*): Cf. KM 2:620–623; SP 408. ‖ "vitriol": "which is a type of *qalqantos*" add. א. 12 "Safflower seed" (QRṬM): Cf. IĞ 876; SHS 1:209, 222 (Ḥet 1, 22). ‖ "It ... stomach": "It is hot, it is good for mange; it makes the menstrual blood flow; it causes a miscarriage and prevents the sperm from being fertile" א. ‖ "dry": "it softens the stool" O. 13 "Tar (or liquid pitch)" (QṬR'N): Cf. SHS 1:387–388 (Ayin 15); "Tar ... fertile": Om. א. ‖ "hot": "very hot" O. 14 "Saltwort" (Q'QLY): Cf. IĞ 466.

15 קרטאס הוא עלים עשויים מן האגמים לבן כששורפין אותו יועיל אפרו משפיעת דם ויכנס בפדלקונים.

16 קצב אלדרירה ב״מ קנים: יש בו קרירות וקביצות.

17 קפר ובלעז אישפלטום היהודי גנאגום(?): חם רך.

18 קלב וב״מ לב הוא זרע לבן הודיי ונקרא כן מפני שהוא דומה ללב כל ב״ח: יגיר השתן ויפרך החצץ.

19 קצב אלדרירה ובלעז קלאמוש ארומאטיגא וב״מ קנה בושם: חם טוב לאצטומכה ולכבד כשיחובש בו.

אות הריש

1 רוסכתג בלעז קוברי ארש או פרט לטי׳ אאישאו שיתום וב״מ נחשת שרוף: יצביע השער ויגליד השחין וישלשל המים.

2 ראונד ובלעז ראיש ברברש: חם טוב לכבד והאצטומכה והמכה כשישתה.

3 ראתינג ובלעז דאגה דפין וב״ח שרף האסטרובלין: יצמיח הבשר ויכנס ברטיות.

4 ראזיאנג ובלעז פנוייל: יגיר השתן ויועיל מן הקדחות הישנות והלח ממנו ירבה החלב בשדים ויחדד הראות כשכוחלין בו.

---

15 קרטאס ... בפדלקונים: om. O || הוא עלים עשויים מן האגמים לבן: om. ב || בפדלקונים: בפלדקונים א 16 אלדרירה: אלדרי א קצב ... וקביצות: om. O 17 קפר ובלעז אישפלטום היהודי גנאגום(?): חם רך: om. O 18 וב״מ לב הוא זרע לבן הודיי ונקרא כן מפני שהוא דומה ללב כל ב״ח: om. ב

1 רוסכתג: רוסתג הוא קרקוש א 2 ראונד: ראויד א || והאצטומכה: والسقطة add. O 3 האסטרובלין: حارّ add. O 4 פנוייל: حارّ add. O

15 Paper; i.e., sheets prepared from reeds (papyrus); [it is] white: When it is burned the ashes are beneficial for bleedings; it is also [good when it is] used as part of enemas.

16 Cane (reed); Rabb. Hebr. QNYM: It is cold and astringent.

17 Bitumen; Rom.–Hebr. ʾYŠPLṬWM HYHWDY (bitumen of the Jews) GNʾGWM(?): It is hot [and] fine.

18 Common gromwell (*Lithospermum officinale*); Rabb. Hebr. LB; it is a white seed from India; it is called with this name because it is similar to the heart of all living beings: It makes the urine flow and pulverizes [intestinal] stones.

19 Lemongrass (*Cymbopogon Martinii*, or *Cymbopogon citratus*); QLʾMWŠ ʾRWMʾṬYGʾ; Rabb. Hebr. QNH BWŠM: It is hot [and] good for the stomach and liver when it is applied as a poultice to them.

Resh

1 Burned copper; Rom. QWBRY ʾRŠ, or PRṬ; Latin: ʾʾYŠʾW ŠYTWM; Rabb. Hebr. NḤŠT ŠRWP: It [is good for] dyeing the hair; it lets an abscess cicatrize and purges the humors.

2 Chinese rhubarb (*Rheum palmatum var. tanguticum*); Rom. RʾYŠ BRBRŠ: It is hot [and] good for the liver, for the stomach, and for a blow, when it is ingested.

3 Resin (from the pine tree); Rom. DʾGH DPYN; Rabb. Hebr. ŠRP HʾSṬRWBLYN: It regenerates flesh and is [useful when it is] used in plasters.

4 Fennel (*Foeniculum vulgare*); Rom. PNWYYL: It makes the urine flow and is beneficial for chronic fevers; fresh [fennel] increases the mothermilk, and it sharpens vision when it is used as an eye-salve.

---

15 "Paper" (QRṬʾS): Cf. D 2:331; "Paper … enemas": Om. O. ‖ "i.e., sheets prepared from reeds (papyrus); [it is] white": Om. ב. ‖ "enemas" (Hebr. PDLQWNYM): For this unidentified term, see SHS 1:421–422 (Pe 36). 16 "Cane (reed)" (QSB): Cf. DT 1:54; "Cane … astringent": Om. O. 17 "Bitumen" (QPR): Cf. D 2:383; "Bitumen … fine": Om. O. ‖ "(bitumen of the Jews)": Cf. IĞ 380: "Judean asphalt." 18 "Common gromwell" (QLB; i.e., Arab. *qulb*): Cf. IĞ 824. ‖ "Rabb. Hebr. LB … beings": Om ב. 19 "Lemongrass" (QSB ʾLDRYRH): Cf. IĞ 846; SHS 1:450 (Qof 5).

1 "Burned copper" (RWSKTG): Cf. KM 1:594–598; SHS 1:351 (Nun 29). 2 "Chinese rhubarb": Cf. DT 3:2; SP 321. ‖ "stomach": "and for a fall" add. O. 3 "Resin (from the pine tree)" (RʾTYNG): Cf. IĞ 870. ‖ "HʾSṬRWBLYN": "It is hot" add O. 4 "Fennel" (RʾZYʾNG): Cf. IĞ 662; SHS 1:504 (Shin 13).

5 רמאד ובלעז סירנא וב״מ אפר: חם יבש שורף ממסמס המורסות הגסות ורוחץ וביחוד דשן התאנה ויש בו יבשות.

6 רטבה: חמה רטובה וזרעה מוסיף בשכבת הזרע והחלב ומנעימה הגוף.

7 רתה: חמה טובה לעקיצת העקרב כשתשתה ממנו ביין או שינתן ממנו בנחירים. (7)

אות השין

1 שיאף אלמראיר: כבר קדם זכרו.

2 שיאף מאמיתה: חם טוב למורסות החמות כשיוטח בו.

3 שקאקל ובלעז שן שלמון: חם רך מעורר תאות המשגל ומרבה המים.

4 שבאבד: חם טוב לריר הנגר מן הנערים ויועיל מן הכפיון.

5 שילם ובלעז גוליום וב״מ תמכה: חם ממשמש המורסות ומשקיט אותן.

6 שיטרג ובלעז קבשיא וב״מ עדל: חם חד טוב לבהק הלבן והצרעת כשיוטח בו בחומץ.

---

5 הגסות: الرهلة O || ורוחץ וביחוד דשן התאנה ויש בו יבשות: om. O 6 רטובה: ב om. O || ומנעימה הגוף: om. O 7 רתה: emend. ed. רקה אב || או: وللقوة O

1 שיאף אלמראיר: כבר קדם זכרו: om. O || אלמראיר: ב om. 2 מאמיתה: מאמית א 4 שבאבד: شابك O שבאבד ... הכפיון: ב om. || מן: أفواه O add. 5 גוליום: emend. ed. גיליום א || תמכה: emend. ed. תמרה א || ומשקיט אותן: om. O

5 Ashes; Rom. SYRN’; Rabb. Hebr. ’PR: They are hot [and] dry; they burn and dissolve hard tumors [and] have a cleansing effect, especially the ashes of a fig; they also have a drying property.

6 Lucerne (*Medicago sativa*): It is hot and fresh; its seed increases the sperm and the mothermilk and fattens the body.

7 Nickernut (*Caesalpinia Bonduc*): It is hot [and] good for scorpion stings when it is ingested in wine and for facial paresis when it is taken as an errhine.

Shin

1 A collyrium of bile: It has already been mentioned (cf. Mem 17 above).

2 Horned poppy (*Glaucium cornulatum*, or *Glaucium flavum*) collyrium: It is hot [and] good for inflamed tumors when it is rubbed on them.

3 Parsnip (*Pastinaca sekakul*, or *Malabaila secacul*); Rom. ŠN ŠLMWN: It is hot [and] fine; it arouses the sexual lust and increases the humors.

4 ŠB’BK (read: Š’BNK) (*Conyza odora Forsk.*, synonym: *Pluchea dioscoridis*): It is hot [and] good for the spittle that streams from the mouth of children and for epilepsy.

5 Darnel (*Lolium temulentum*); Rom. GWLYWM; Rabb. Hebr. TMKH: It is hot; it dissolves tumors and alleviates [their pain].

6 Pepperweed (*Lepidium latifolium*) or garden cress (*Lepidium sativum*); Rom. QBŠY’; Rabb. Hebr. ‘DL: It is hot [and] sharp; it is good for white *bahaq* and leprosy when it is rubbed with vinegar on [the spots affected by it].

---

5 “Ashes” (RM’D): Cf. D 1:557. ‖ “hard”: “flabby” O. ‖ “[and] have a cleansing effect, especially the ashes of a fig; they also have a drying property”: Om. O. 6 “Lucerne” (RṬBH): Cf. IĞ 913. ‖ “and fresh”: I.e., Arab. *raṭba* refers to to the fresh kind of “lucerne,” while *fiṣfiṣa* refers to the dry kind; the term is missing in O. ‖ “and fattens the body”: Om. O. ‖ “fattens” (מנעימה): Cf. Ḥet 9 above. 7 “Nickernut” (RTH): Cf. IĞ 130. ‖ “and for facial paresis when”: Translated according to O: وللقوة.

1 “collyrium” (ŠY’P): Cf. FAQ 272–274. 2 “Horned poppy” (SY’P M’MYTH): Cf. DT 3:81. 3 “Parsnip” (ŠQ’QL): Cf. IĞ 985. 4 “ŠB’BK (read: Š’BNK)”: I.e., Arab. شابنك; cf. D 1:714; IBF 1273; “ŠB’BK … epilepsy”: Om. ב. ‖ “from the mouth of”: Translated according to O: أفواه. 5 “Darnel” (ŠYLM): Cf. IĞ 998; SHS 1:531 (Tav 6). ‖ “and alleviates [their pain]”: Om. O. 6 “Pepperweed” (ŠYṬRG): Cf. IĞ 33; SHS 1:399–400 (Ayin 39). ‖ “white *bahaq*”: Cf. Ḥet 3 above.

7 שברם ובלעז אישולא או טיטמאל: חם ישלשל בחזקה המרה הכרכומית והלחה הלבנה והוא רע לכבד.

8 שאדנה ובלעז לאפיש אמאטיטש: קר קובץ יבש ינגב הלחות והדמעה מן העין.

9 שב ובלעז אלום: חזק הקביצות יאסוף השנים המתנועעות.

10 שכאע ובלעז קלקא טריפה: חם מועיל מן הקדחות הישנות.

11 שאתרג ובלעז פומוש טירא ובל״ח ⟨שר⟩ הירקות: חם טוב לגרב והחכוך וישלשל המעים.

12 שחם ובלעז שאוי החלב: כלם ממסמסים מרככים דשנים מזהימים וכל שכן חלבי הכליות.

13 שקורדיון הוא השום המדברי: חם טוב לעובי הטחול ולהטפת השתן והחצץ.

14 שקאיק אלנעמן ובלעז רושילש ובל״ח שושנת המלך: חם לוטש חשכת העין ולובנו ויכנס בשחרות השער.

15 שוניז ובלעז גיט ובל״מ קצח: חם חריף יתיך הליחה ⟨הלבנה⟩ ויוריד הזיכום ויגרש הרוחות.

16 שנכאר: חם טוב לבהק כשיוטח בו נילוש בחומץ ויועיל לירקון כשישתה ולעובי הטחול.

---

7 בחזקה: om. ב || הלבנה: والما add. O 8 שאדנה: שאדנג א || קובץ: om. O || ינגב הלחות והדמעה מן העין: يدخل في الأكحال O 10 שכאע: شكاعى O 11 שאתרג: שאדנג א 12 דשנים מזהימים וכל שכן חלבי הכליות: om. O 13 ולהטפת השתן והחצץ: om. O 15 חריף: om. O || ויוריד: emend. ed. ויורד א 16 שנכאר: emend. ed. שיבאר אב || נילוש בחומץ: om. O || הטחול: وهو حجر معقف يحمل من عمان add. O

7 Quacksalver's spurge (*Euphorbia Pithyusa*); Rom. 'YŠWL', or ṬYṬM'L: It is hot; it purges the yellow bile and the phlegm with force; it is bad for the liver.

8 Hematite; Rom. L'PYŠ 'M'ṬYṬŠ: It is cold, astringent, [and] dry; it dries the moisture and a continous weeping discharge (rhyas) in the eye.

9 Alum; Rom. 'LWM: It is very astringent, [and] it holds back teeth from moving.

10 Thistle; Rom. QLQ' ṬRYPH: It is hot [and] beneficial for chronic fevers.

11 Fumitory (*Fumaria officinalis*); Rom. PWMWŠṬYR'; Rabb. Hebr. [ŠR] HYRQWT: It is hot [and] good for mange and for itch; it purges the intestines.

12 Fat; Rom. Š'WY [Rabb. Hebr.] HḤLB: All [kinds of] fat dissolve and soften; they are fat and unwholesome, especially [the fat] in the intestines.

13 Water germander (*Teucrium scordium*); i.e., wild garlic: It is hot [and] good for a thick spleen and for dribbling urine and [intestinal] stones.

14 Poppy anemone (*Anemone coronaria*, or broad-leaved anemone [*Anemone hortensis*]); Rom. RWŠYLŠ; Rabb. Hebr. ŠWŠNT HMLK: It is hot; it cures dimsightedness and leucoma and [is good when it] is used to blacken the hair.

15 Black cumin (*Nigella sativa*); Rom. GYṬ; Rabb. Hebr. QṢḤ: It is hot [and] sharp; it dissolves the phlegm, stops a catarrh, and dispels winds.

16 Alkanet (*Alkanna tinctoria*): It is hot; it is good for *bahaq* when it is mixed with vinegar and then rubbed on it; it is beneficial for jaundice and for a thick (enlarged) spleen when it is ingested.

---

7 "Quacksalver's spurge" (ŠBRM): Cf. IĞ 425, 777. || "'YŠWL', or ṬYṬM'L": See Gerrit Bos and Guido Mensching, "A 15th Century medico-botanical synonym list (Ibero-Romance-Arabic) in Hebrew characters," *Panace@*, 7, no. 24 (2006): 266. || "phlegm": "and the [other] humors" add. O. 8 "Hematite (Š'DNH); Rom. L'PYŠ 'M'ṬYṬŠ": Cf. KM 2:719–726; M 369; Berakhyah Ben Natronai ha-Nakdan, *Sefer Ko'ah ha-Avanim* (*On the Virtue of Stones*): *With a lexicological analysis of the Romance terminology and source study*, eds. Gerrit Bos and Julia Zwink (Leiden: Brill, 2010), pp. 118–119 (no. 9). || "astringent": Om. O. || "it dries the moisture and a continous weeping discharge (rhyas) in the eye": "it is [beneficial when it is] used as an eye-salve" O. || "a continuous weeping discharge (rhyas)" (דמעה): Cf. Bet 11. 9 "Alum" (ŠB): Cf. KM 2:726–729; SHS 1:308 (Mem 10). 10 "Thistle" (ŠK''): The term *šukā'ā* was used for a group of thistle species, especially Scotch thistle, *Onopordum acanthium*, and perhaps also plume thistle, *Cirsium ferox*; cf. IĞ 12. 11 "Fumitory" (Š'TRG): Cf. IĞ 138; SHS 1:522 (Shin 50). 12 "Fat" (ŠḤM): Cf. D 1:732. || "they are fat and unwholesome, especially [the fat] in the intestines": Om. O. 13 "Water germander" (ŠQWRDYWN): Cf. IĞ 45; SHS 1:505–506 (Shin 16). || "and for dribbling urine and [intestinal] stones": Om. O. 14 "Poppy anemone": Cf. IĞ 613; SHS 1:508 (Shin 20). || "cures dimsightedness": Cf. Mem 17 above. 15 "Black cumin" (ŠWNYZ): Cf. IĞ 364; SHS 1:457 (Qof 17). 16 "Alkanet" (SNK'R): Cf. DT 4:23. || "*bahaq*": Cf. Zayin 2 above. || "mixed with vinegar and then": Om. O. || "it is a deformed stone that is brought from Oman": Add. O.

אות התו

1 תודרי: חם מוסיף בתאות המשגל.

2 תותיה: חמה וחזקה להפסקת ריח האצילים.

3 תרבד ובלעז תרביד: חם רך ישלשל הלחה התפלה והלחה הלבנה.

4 תרנגבין ובלעז מאנה וב״מ ⟨מן⟩: דק שוה ירפה המעים ויאות לכל טבע.

5 תמר הנדי ובלע׳ תמראינדי: קר משלשל ומשבר המרה הכרכומית והדם.

6 תאפסיא ובלעז טאפסיא: חמה מאד תצמיח השער במדוה השועל ותועיל כשמושכין בה את הגוף מן הרפיון.

7 תיל ובלעז אגורשטש אגרם וב״ח חצב: יגיר השתן ויפרד החצץ.

---

1 תודרי: תותבר א ‖ בתאות המשגל: בשכבת הזרע ב 2 חמה וחזקה להפסקת ריח האצילים: جيد لتقوية العين قاطع للصنان O 3 הלחה התפלה והלחה הלבנה: البلغم O 4 דק: om. O ‖ ויאות לכל טבע: om. O 5 הנדי: om. א ‖ משלשל ומשבר המרה הכרכומית: ملين البطن يقمع الصفرا O

Tav

1 Hedgemustard (*Sisymbrium officinale*): It is hot [and] increases sexual lust.
2 Zinc oxide: It is hot and a strong ingredient to stop armpit odor.
3 Turpeth (*Operculina turpethum*, synonym: *Ipomoea turpethum*): It is hot [and] fine; it purges the crude phlegm.
4 Manna (the sugary concretions on certain desert plants, especially diverse species of *Astragalus*); Rom. M'NH; Rabb. Hebr. [MN]: It is fine [and] moderate; it softens the stools and is good for every nature (constitution).
5 Tamarind (*Tamarindus indica*); Rom. TMR'YNDY: It is cold; it purges and checks the yellow bile and the blood.
6 Thapsia (*Thapsia garganica*); Rom. Ṭ'PSY': It is very hot; it makes the hair grow when someone suffers from alopecia, and it is beneficial for feebleness when it is rubbed on the body.
7 Bermuda grass (*Cynodon dactylon*); Rom. 'GWRŠṬŠ 'GRM; Rabb. Hebr. ḤṢB: It makes the urine flow and pulverizes [intestinal] stones.

1 "Hedgemustard" (TWDRY): Cf. IĞ 1005. || "sexual lust": "sperm" ב. 2 "Zinc oxide" (TWTYH): Cf. KM 1:361–369. || "It is hot and a strong ingredient to stop armpit odor": Cf. O: "It is good for strengthening the eyes [and for] stopping armpit odor." 3 "Turpeth" (TRBD): Cf. DT 4:121, n. 4. || "the crude phlegm": "the phlegm" O. 4 "Manna" (TRNGBYN): Cf. M 386. || "fine [and]": Om. O. || "and is good for every nature (constitution)": Om. O. 5 "Tamarind" (TMR HNDY): Cf. IĞ 805. || "it purges and checks the yellow bile": "it softens the stools and checks the yellow bile" O. || "checks": Translated after O: يقمع; Shem Tov reads, "breaks." 6 "Thapsia" (T'PSY'): Cf. IĞ 433; SHS 1:202–203 (Zayin 10). 7 "Bermuda grass (TYL); Rom. 'GWRŠṬŠ 'GRS; Rabb. Hebr. ḤṢB": Cf. SHS 1:219–220 (Ḥet 17).

Supplement: Romance and Latin Terms in the *Sefer Almansur*

Preliminary Note

Below we list the Romance (mostly Old Occitan) and Latin terms that appear in the text and give a short explanation for each of them, mostly with the aim of identifying the language at issue, the meaning of the term, and its documentation in other texts.[1] In this preliminary note, we briefly point out some features of this language that are visible in the relevant lexical items.[2] Like the languages of the Iberian Peninsula and French, Occitan displays the shift from Latin intervocalic -T- to *-d-*, as part of the so-called Western Romance lenition. This can be seen in the feminine participle ending *-ada* (< Lat. -ATA) in *muscada* (מושקדא—MWŠQD', Gimel 10). We can exclude French, which lost this *-d-* (yielding *musquée*), whereas Italian, an Eastern Romance language, has conserved the Latin -T- (see *noce moscata* for "nutmeg").[3] Words like *encens*, 'frankincense' (אנשנש—'NŠNŠ, Kaf 9) or *foc* "fire" (פוג—PWG, Nun 7), from Lat. INCENSUM and FOCUM, respectively, show the complete loss of the Latin ending -UM,[4] so that we can exclude Spanish, where the ending is preserved as a final *-o* (*incienso* and *fuego*).[5] These examples also show that stressed Latin Ĕ and Ŏ are maintained as *e* and *o* in Occitan instead of becoming diphthongs as in Spanish.

The properties mentioned so far also apply to Catalan, a language that is very similar to Occitan. Recall that Shem Tov originally came from Tortosa in Catalonia, so that we have to suppose that Catalan was his mother tongue. However, in most cases in which Occitan is different from Catalan, Shem Tov rather used

1 We would like to thank Britta Gemmeke for helping us to localize the Romance and Latin terms in dictionaries and other documents.

2 For more detailed descriptions of characteristics of Old Occitan and for references, cf. Bos et al., *Medical Synonym Lists, Part 1*, pp. 32–52; Cyril Aslanov, "Occitan," in: Mensching and Savelsberg, *Manual*; Guido Mensching, "Eléments lexicaux et textes occitans"; Guido Mensching and Julia Zwink, "L'ancien occitan en tant que langage scientifique."

3 Note, by the way, that Shem Tov uses a hybrid Hebrew–Romance compound term for 'nutmeg': אגוז מושקדא—'GWZ MWŠQD'. This is the only example of this kind in the text. For the more frequent use of Latin–Romance compounds, see below.

4 Most Romance words derive from the Latin accusative forms.

5 The same holds for Portuguese but not for Catalan.

the Occitan form. For example,[6] Latin intervocalic -D- was lost in Catalan, but preserved in Occitan: Lat. CODA > Catalan *coa*, but Occitan *coda* ("tail"); see entry Dalet 10, where we have קודא (QWD'). The so-called "n-mobile" of certain Occitan words, resulting mostly from Latin secondary final N, is present in Shem Tov's Romance lexemes, while it generally disappeared in Catalan. Examples are Old Occitan *jassemin*, "jasmine" (ישמין—YŠMYN, Bet 10) vs. Old Catalan *gessimí* or Old Occitan *pin*, "pine tree" (פין—PYN, Resh 3). The Latin diphthong -AU- is preserved in Occitan, whereas it monophthongized to *-o-* in Catalan; see מברילה (MBRYLH, Ayin 4), which is the Old Occitan *maurel(h)a*, "nightshade" (vs. Old Catalan *morella*). Finally, we find several lexemes that are typically Occitan and do not exist in Catalan: נשטורש (NŠṬWRŠ, Het 8), the plural of Old Occitan *nazitor(t)* "garden cress" (vs. Catalan *morritort*); לויאמי (LWY'MY, Kaf 18), Occitan *levame*, "leaven" (vs. Old Catalan *llevat*); and רומזי (RWMZY, Ayin 9), Old Occitan *romeze*, "common brumble" (vs. Old Catalan *romeguera*).

There are, however, extremely few examples of words in the *Sefer Almansur* that are only documented in Old Catalan, but not in Old Occitan. We were able to identify **peix de saget* (PYŠ DŠYYṬ, entry Samekh 2), documented in Old Catalan as *peix saget*, "arrow fish"; note that the variant *saget* ("arrow") is exclusively Catalan and was *sa(g)eta* in Old Occitan. Similarly, *apopònac* ('PWPWNQ, Gimel 2), "resin of Opopanax," seems to be Old Catalan and not Old Occitan (*opoponac*). These isolated items can be interpreted as an influence of Shem Tov's mother tongue Catalan.

[Bet 6] פוליפודיאו—PWLYPWDY'W: Lat. *polipodiu[m]* for Polypodium vulgare L. (cf. SHS 1:368–369, Samekh 32).

[Bet 7] בלבוס—BLBWS: Lat. *bulbus*, "bulb of every kind of plant," and, according to the *Alphita*, especially "bulb of Narcissus pseudo-narcissus L." (GGA 376). BLBWS may also transcribe Arab. *bulbūs*, "bulb of Muscari comosum Mill. or other plants" (cf. MBG 16).

[Bet 8] קורויולא או קורגיולא—QWRWYWL' or QWRGYWL': Romance, probably O. Occ. *correiola*, or O. Cat. *corriola* / O. Occ. *corrigiola* or O. Cat. *corretjola* for Convolvulus arvensis L. (cf. SHS 1:461, Qof 23).

[Bet 9] אוזימו גירופלא—'WZYMW GYRWPL': The compound term is related to **ozimum gariofilatum*, which is used in Ms Munich, Bayer. Staatsbibl. 87 (fol. 128ʳ) as an equivalent of Arab. *ifranǧamušk* (افرنجمشك), a variant of

6 For phenomenons that distinguish Occitan from Catalan, cf. Bos, Hussein, Mensching, and Savelsberg, *Medical Synonym Lists, Part 1*, pp. 39–41.

baranǧamušk (برنجمشك), designating a type of mint, perhaps Ocimum minimum L. (cf. BKM; DT 3:43).

[Bet 10] ישמין—YŠMYN: Probably O. Occ *jassemin*, "jasmine" (Jasminum fructicans L.) (FEW 19:199a).

[Bet 13] שליום—ŠLYWM: Lat. *psyllium*, "fleawort" (Plantago psyllium L.) (NPRA 210); the term appears in the same transcription in IT 22.3, 27.3.

[Bet 14] אנוש קאשטוש—'NWŠ Q'ŠṬWŠ: Lat. *agnus castus*, "monk's pepper" (Vitex agnus castus L.) (cf. SHS 1:114–115, Alef 30).

[Bet 15] קמומילא—QMWMYL': Late Lat., O. Occ. or O. Cat. *camomilla* for "chamomile" (Anthemis arvensis L.) (cf. SHS 1:456–457, Qof 15).

[Gimel 1] בומיטא—BWMYṬ': Probably Romance or a Romanized variant *vomita* of Lat. *vomica*, abbreviated variant of *nux vomica*, "vomic nut" (Strychnos nux-vomica L.) (GGA 490). The compound NWS BWMṬY (Mss PO) appears in the SHS 2, Nun 1, where it is interpreted as a mixed Latin–Romance compound **nos vomiti*. Cf. also SHS 1:102, Alef 15, for NWS BWMYQ' (Ms P), transcribing O. Occ. **nos vomica*, id.

[Gimel 2] אפופונק—'PWPWNQ: Probably O. Cat. *apopònac* (DCVB 1:781a), "resin of Opopanax chrironium Koch.," borrowing of Latin *opopanax* (Sin 110, fn. 22). For O. Occ., only *opoponac* is documented (PSW 5:496b). Cf. also SHS 2, Alef 66: 'PWPNQ and IT 10.5, etc.: 'PWPWNQ.

[Gimel 3] פוליום מונטנום—PWLYWM MWNṬNWM: Late Lat. *polium montanum* for Teucrium Polium L. (cf. SHS 1:363–364, Samekh 20).

[Gimel 4] גנסיאנה—GNSY'NH: Lat. *gentiana* (MLWB 4:669), or O. Occ. *gensiana* / O. Cat. *genciana*, "gentian" (Gentiana lutea L.) (RMA 172; AdV 482, etc.). Cf. also SHS 2, Gimel 4: GNSY'N' and IT 10.3, etc.: GYNSY'N'.

[Gimel 5] גיף—GYP: O. Occ. *gip* for "gypsum" (cf. SHS 1:152, Gimel 10).

[Gimel 7] בלאושטיאש—BL'WŠṬY'Š: Plural of O. Occ./ O. Cat. *balaustia*, "blossom of the wild pomegranate tree" (Punica granatum L.) (cf. SHS 1:338, Nun 4).

[Gimel 8] סיטול—SYṬWL: Probably O. Occ. / O. Cat. *citoal*, "curcuma root" (Curcuma zedoaria) (FEW 19:202b; DCVB 3:175b); cf. also SHS 2, Ayin 2: SYṬWW(')L, id.

[Gimel 9] קשטור—QŠṬWR: Romance, possibly O. Fr. *castor*, "secretion found in the body of beaver, used in medicine, castoreum" (FEW 2:474b). Also cf. Lat. / O. Occ. *castoreum* and O. Occ. *castorea*, id. (MLWB 2:344; FEW l.c.; LR 2:355b).

[Gimel 10] אגוז מושקדא—'GWZ MWŠQD': Bilingual Hebr.—O. Occ. compound, i.e., Hebr. 'GWZ ("nut"), and O. Occ. *muscada*, the whole term corresponding to O. Occ. *nos muscada*, "nutmeg" (Myristica fragrans Houtt.) (DAO 631).

[Gimel 11] אגריק—'GRYQ: O. Occ. or O. Cat. *agaric*(*h*), "genus of mushrooms of the Agaricaceae family that includes various species growing on the trunks of certain trees" (DCVB 1:278b; DAO 1008); cf. also SHS 2, Alef 2: 'GRYQ and IT 18.3, etc.: id.

[Gimel 12] נאשקא או ח(א)ריבברא—N'SQ' or Ḥ('?)RYBBR': It is unclear why the author identifies Arab. גאפת ("agrimony," Agrimonia eupatoria L.) with Romance N'SQ', which may be related to O. Gasc. *nasca*, Inula viscosa, Pulicaria viscosa (DAO 1069; FEW 21:178b). The second synonym Ḥ('?)RYBBR' could not be identified; initial Ḥet indicates that the term is not Romance.

[Gimel 13] גלוט—GLWṬ: Probably O. Occ. *glut*, "viscous matter, gum; kind of make-up" (FEW 4:169b). The O. Cat. word is *gluten*, id. (cf. DCVB 6:322a).

[Gimel 14] שלזין—ŠLZYN: Romance, probably a non-documented O. Occ. variant **salzin* for "variety of willow" (Salix L.). The usual O. Occ. word for "willow" was *sals*, *sauze*, next to others (cf. FEW 11:100b), but note that in Old Franco-Provençal variants like *saucin*, "willow," are attested; in M. French *sauzin* is documented for "a kind of olive" (FEW 11:101b). Cf. also. ŠLZY, id., in SHS 1:388–389, Ayin 16.

[Gimel 15] לורוש—LWRWŠ: Lat. *laurus* for "laurel" (Laurus nobilis L.) (NPRA 40; NGH 2:589); cf. also SHS 2, Lamed 2: LWRWŠ and IT 30.4: L'BRWŠ, among others.

[Dalet 2] לורדמוני—LWRDMWNY: The Romance term (**laur dam*(*p*)*ne*?), probably meaning "oleander" (Nerium oleander L.), actually contains two words: the first three letters (LWR) correspond to O. Occ. *laur* / O. Cat. *llaur*, "laurel;" DMWNY is a variant that belongs to the Greek δάφνη, which often appears with a parasitic *-m-* in Medieval Latin (e.g., *dampnis*, "laurel," in the *Alphita* (D7), GGA 406). Cf. the explanation of the term in the same spelling in SHS 1:182–183, He 3.

[Dalet 3] וישק—WYŠQ: Romance (O. Occ. / O. Cat.) *visc*(*h*), *vesc* for "mistle" (Viscum album L.) and "bird-lime," since the lime was from the sticky sap of the mistle berries (DAO 1173; FEW 14:523b; DCVB 10:837a).

[Dalet 5] פושטא—PWŠṬ': Probably Romance (O. Occ. / O. Cat.) *fusta* for "wood, tree" (DAO 449–2; FEW 3:915b; DCVB 6:103b). The Hebrew synonym suggests the reading "plane tree" (Platanus orientalis), whose O. Occ. name was *platani* (DAO 500; FEW 9:36b), the O. Cat. *plàtan* (DCVB 8:653b).

[Dalet 8] שנג דראגין—ŠNG DR'GYN: The letter yod is probably misspelled for waw. O. Occ. documented variants of this term are *sanc de drag*(*u*)*on* / *sang de draguo*(*n*) / *sanch de drago*, "dark red resin, produced by different exotic plants, in particular by the Calamus draco, used in medicine as adstringent"

(DAO 569); cf. SHS 1:168, Dalet 2. The corresponding Cat. term (*sanch de dragó*) is only documented since the sixteenth century (DCVB 9:724a).

[Dalet 9] קנטרידש—QNṬRYDŠ: Lat. *cantharides*, nom. or acc. plural of *cantharis* or the plural of Cat. *cantàrida* (attested since ca. 1450). There is no documentation of a corresponding word in O. Occ.; cf. SHS 1:311, Mem 16; and IT 18.4.

[Dalet 10] קודא דקאבל—QWD' DQ'BL: O. Occ. **coda de caval*(*h*), literally meaning "horse-tail," probably designating diverse species of plants of the genus Equisetum; cf. SHS 1:199, Zayin 4, and SHS 2, Qof 10.

[Dalet 11] אור—'WR: O. Occ. or O. Cat. *aur*, "gold"; cf. SHS 1:155–156, Gimel 15.

[He 1] מירבולנש אינדיש—MYRBWLNŠ 'YNDYŠ: O. Occ or O. Cat. **mirabolans indis* for "Indian myrobalans"; cf. SHS 1:186, He 8.

[He 4] איבוקושטידום—'YBWQWŠṬYDWM: Accusative singular of Late Lat. *hypoquistidus*, "hypocist" (Cytinus hypocistis L.); cf. SHS 1:360, Samekh 12, where the term figures in its nominative form 'YBWQWŠṬYDWS.

[He 5] אנפסק—'NPSQ, or ארבה פורבאדה—'RBH PWRB'DH: The second synonym is probably a romanized variant of M. Lat. *herba perforata*, "St. John's wort" (Hypericum perforatum L.) (GGA 445), i.e., **herba perforada* (cf. SHS 2, Alef 70). The first synonym 'NPSQ could not be identified.

[Zayin 1] זינגברי—ZYNGBRY: **Zingebre*, "ginger" (Zingiber officinalis Roscoe), seems to be a Romance loanword of Lat. *zingiber*. The usual O. Occ. and O. Cat. term is *gingebre*, with variants *zimzembre*, *gingibre*, *gengibre*, *gengebre*, among others (cf. FEW 14:663b; DCVB 6:289b–290a); see also SHS 2, Gimel 8.

[Zayin 2]: ארישטולוגיאה לונגא—ARYŠṬWLWGY'H LWNG', and ארישטולוגיא רדונדא—ARYŠṬWLWGY' RDWND': The two compounds represent the two types of *aristolochia*, "birthwort" (Aristolochia L.): The first one is Lat. *aristologia longa*, "long aristolochia" (MLWB 1:954), for which no O. Occ. or O. Cat. loan translations are known to us.[7] The second one is O. Occ. / O. Cat. *aristologia redonda*, "round aristolochia" (DAO Suppl. 1137, AdV 478). Cf. IT 30.4, 30.5; and SHS 2, Alef 33.

[Zayin 3] איזופוש—'YZWPWŠ, or איזוף—'YZWP: The first term is Lat. (*h*)*yssopus* or *ysopus*, *isopus* for Hyssopus officinalis L. The Romance synonym transcribes O. Occ. / O. Cat. *isop* or *ysop* with the same meaning (DAO 1070; DCVB 6:728a); cf. SHS 2, Alef 34 and Mem 10.

7 O. Sp. *aristologia luenga*, id. (DETEMA 1:146a) is the only Romance attestation.

[Zayin 5] ארגימנט—'RGYMNṬ, or ויטרייול—WYṬRYYWL: The same synonymy is given in SHS 1:454–455, Qof 11.[8] 'RGYMNṬ should correspond, according to the Hebrew synonym, to O. Occ. *airamen*, "black liquid, ink; vitriol," or O. Occ. / O. Cat. *atrament*, "vitriol" (also cf. DOM 5:396a, *airamen*). It seems to be corrupt or might be contaminated by O. Occ. / O. Cat. *a*(*i*)*gramen*(*t*), "sourly," because sulfate (vitriol) is sour. The second term is O. Occ. *vetriol* or O. Occ. / O. Cat. *vitriol* for "sulfate," which was used in the production of ink.

[Zayin 6] ארגינט ביב—'RGYNṬ BYB: O. Occ. / O. Cat. *argent viu* for "mercury" (DCVB 1:853a–855a; DAO 363); cf. SHS 2, Alef 92.

[Zayin 7] אורפימנט—'WRPYMNṬ: O. Occ. / O. Cat. *aurpi*(*g*)*men*(*t*) or *orpiment* for "natural arsenic sulfide;" cf. SHS 1:353, Samekh 2.

[Zayin 8] אשפומא דמר—'ŠPWM' DMR: Romance (O. Occ. or O. Cat.) **espuma de mar*, literally "sea foam." For *espuma* "foam," cf. FEW (12:214a); DCVB (5:459a); for *mar*, "sea," FEW (6.1:317a); DCVB (7:225b). Also cf. SHS 1:228, Ḥet 33 (**escuma marina*, id.).

[Zayin 10] אלפלור דסנמומי—'LPLWR DSNMWMY: Romance for "blossom of cinnamon." The O. Occ. / O. Cat. compound expression PLWR DSNMWMY, *flor de cinamomi*, also figures in SHS 1:434, Zade 9. It appears here with the prefix 'L-, which should be interpreted as the Arabic definite article *al*-.

[Zayin 11] ווירדיט—WWYRDYṬ: O. Occ. / O. Cat. *verdet* for "verdigris" or "cupric carbonate or acetate and other similar matters which arise from humidity"; cf. SHS 1:406–407, Pe 11.

[Zayin 12] וירמליון—WYRMLYWN: O. Occ. *vermelhon* "red makeup"; cf. SHS 1:255, Samekh 4.

[Ḥet 1] אממו—'MMW: M. Lat. *amomum* with the lack of final *-m*, typical for medieval Hebrew texts (cf. SHS 1:46–47).[9] The term was used for designating several odoriferous plants (cf. FEW 24:463b). For O. Occ., the term *amo* is documented (FEW loc. cit.), and for O. Cat., *amomi*, prob. from the Lat. genitive as used in recipes (DCVB 1:635b); cf. SHS 2, Alef 26.

[Ḥet 3] גראנא דאינדי—GR'N' D'YNDY: O. Occ. / O. Cat. **grana de indi*/*d'indi* for "kernels of indigo"; cf. SHS 1:150, Gimel 6.

[Ḥet 4] ביבא קורבינא—BYB' QWRBYN': The synonymy of the Arab. and Hebr. terms meaning "houseleek" (Sempervivum tectorum L.) with a Romance

8 'RGYMNṬ, or WYṬRYWL (Ms P).

9 The similarity of the variant to O. Sp. *amomo* (DETEMA 1:100b) or Old Vaudois (= Franco-Provençal) *amomo* (FEW 24:463b) is most probably coincidental.

compound BYB' QWRBYN', **viva corvina*, is also given in the entry SHS 1:211, Ḥet 4. In this entry, the compound could not be identified as a whole, but the first term *viva* is probably related to Lat. *sempervіva*, "houseleek"; the second one might transcribe the Lat. adjective *corvinus* (or a Romance equivalent), which often appears in compound plant names.

[Ḥet 5] קולוקוינטידא—QWLWQWYNṬYD': Late Lat. *coloquinthida*, "colocynth" (Citrullus colocynthis Schrad.). The term was also used in Romance, e.g., O. Occ. *colloquintida* / *coloquintida*; for Cat., *coloquinta* is documented. Cf. SHS 1:220–221, Ḥet 20.

[Ḥet 7] טריבולוס מרינוש—ṬRYBWLWS MRYNWŠ, or אשפונגא מרי—'ŠPWNG' MRY: The first compound term is Lat. *tribulus marinus*, which is, in general, identified with "water caltrop" (Trapa natans L.) (NPRA 263). It also appears in SHS 1:497–498, Shin 4, where it is identified with the same Arab. and Hebr. terms, meaning Tribulus terrestris L. ("caltrop"). Indeed, it should be noticed that the second compound term also refers to a sea organism: 'ŠPWNG' is O. Occ. *esponga* or O. Occ. / O. Cat. *esponja*, "poriferous substance stemming from a marine zoophyte that absorbs liquids, sponge" (FEW 12:207a; DCVB 5:452ab); MRY is the O. Occ. / O. Cat. adjective *mari*, "marine, pertinent to the sea" (FEW 6.1:344a; DCVB 7:247b) figuring here without mobile *-n*. The term as a whole is thus "marine sponge."

[Ḥet 8] נשטורש—NŠṬWRŠ: Plural of O. Occ. *nazitor*(*t*), or *na*(*s*)*sitor*(*t*) for "garden cress" (Lepidum sativum L.); the Cat. word for this plant is *morritort* (cf. SHS 1:503, Shin 12).

[Ḥet 9] אלקינא—'LQYN': Late Lat. *alchanna*, O. Occ. *al*(*a*)*quana* / *alquana*, or O. Cat. *alcanna* / *alquena* for "henna" (Lawsonia inermis L.); cf. SHS 1:275, Kaf 20.

[Ḥet 10] ליסיאום—LYSY'WM: Lat. *licium* / *lycium*, which has two meanings according to NPRA (149): 1. the sap of an oriental buckthorn (e.g., Rhamnus petiolaris, Rh. lycoïdes, Rh. punctata Boiss.); 2. Lycium Indicum, which is the sap extracted from the husk of the Acacia catechu Willd.; cf. SHS 2, Lamed 14; IT 15.3, inter alia. Also cf. entry [Pe 4].

[Ḥet 11] פירי—PYRY: O. Occ. or O. Cat. *ferre* for "iron;" cf. SHS 1:236, Ḥet 49.

[Ṭet 1] רושא קנינא—RWŠ' QNYN': Lat. *rosa canina*, meaning "dog rose" (Rosa canina L.). The term was also common in Romance, e.g., in O. Occ. and O. Cat. medical texts (cf. SHS 1:197–198, Zayin 2).

[Ṭet 2] בול שגלאטום—BWL ŠGL'ṬWM: The compound term is a blend of O. Occ. *bol*(*h*) / O. Cat. *bol*(*l*), "bolus, medical clay," and of Lat. *sigillatum*, "sealed," literally thus "sealed clay"; cf. SHS 1:239–240, Ṭet 1: BWL ŠǦYL'ṬWM (Ms P). Note that Romance *bol* was commonly specified by the adjective *armenic*,

"Armenian" (FEW 25:271b), and that Lat. *sigillatum* usually co-occurs with *terra*, "earth": *terra sigillata*, both terms corresponding to "medical clay" (cf. SHS 1 loc. cit.).

[Ṭet 4] טמריסי—ṬMRYSY: O. Occ. *tamarici*, "tamarisk" (DAO 779); cf. SHS 2, Ṭet 2.

[Ṭet 5] אשפודיאום—'ŠPWDYWM: M. Lat. variant **espodium* of *spodium*, with a prothetic *e-*. During the Middle Ages, it designated several types of ashes, in particular of the roots of certain canes (GGA 546f.); cf. also SHS 2, Alef 39.

[Ṭet 6] לינטילאה—LYNṬYL'H, or לינטילולא—LYNṬYLWL': The first synonym is O. Occ. *lentil(h)a* / *lentilla* or O. Cat. *l(l)entilla* for "lentil"; cf. SHS 1:377–378, Ayin 2. The second term seems to transcribe O. Cat. *llentillola*, a medical plant (DCVB 6:949a). The diminutive suffix *-ol(a)* also existed in O. Occ. (cf. WfP 240ff.), so that we might hypothesize an O. Occ. variant **lentil(h)ola*, "little lentil." In Mod. Provençal, we find *lentihòla* for Lotus corniculatus L. (FEW 5:251b).

[Yod 1] מנדרגולא—MNDRGWL': O. Occ. *mandragolha* / O. Cat. *mandragola*, "mandrake" (Mandragora officinarum L.); cf. SHS 1:169, Dalet 3.

[Yod 2] טיטמאל—ṬYṬM'L, or לשושקלי—LŠWŠQLY: ṬYṬM'L represents O. Occ. / O. Cat. *titimal*, "spurge" (Euphorbia L.); cf. SHS 1:509, Shin 22. The second term is O. Occ. *lachuscla* (Mod. Occ. *lachuscle*), id. (DAO 1140, FEW 5:125a), which does not exist in Cat. Cf. also IT 16.3.

[Kaf 2] כונדוס—KWNDWS: The Romance word **kundus* is an Arabism derived from Arabic *kundus*, meaning "sneezewort" (Achillea ptarmica L.); "hellebore" (Helleborus L.); cf. SHS 1:213, Ḥet 7. For O. Fr., the variants *condise*, *condes*, and *condisi* are attested (AdOr 331).

[Kaf 3] גראנא דטמריס—GR'N' DṬMRYS: The Romance term is O. Occ. *grana de tamaris*, "seed of the tamarisk" (Tamarix articulata Vahl [Tamarix orientalis Forsk.]). For O. Occ. *tamaris*, "tamarisk," cf. SHS 2, Ṭet 2; also cf. entry [Ṭet 2]; for Romance *grana*, cf. entry [Ḥet 3] above.

[Kaf 4] קקברי—QQBRY: M. Lat. *cacabre*, "amber" (GGA 377), loanword from Arab. *kahrabā*; cf. also SHS 2, Qof 21.

[Kaf 5] כאמידריוש—K'MYDRYWŠ: Lat. *camedreos*, meaning Teucrium chamaedrys L., Teucrium lucidum L., Veronica Chamaedrys L., and Stachys officinalis L.; cf. SHS 1:146, Bet 30.

[Kaf 9] אנשנש—'NŠNŠ: O. Occ. or O. Cat. *encens*, "frankincense," i.e., gum resin of diverse Boswellia species (DAO 571; DECLC 3:320b). Cf. SHS 2, Alef 42 and Ṭet 10.

[Kaf 10] קובבש—QWBBŠ: Plural of O. Occ. or O. Cat. *cubeba* (i.e., *cubebas* [-*es*]); for "Cubeb pepper" (Piper cubeba L.), from Arab. *kubbāba* (FEW 19:97a; DAO 1177; DCVB 3:797a); cf. SHS 2, Kaf 1 and Kaf 2.

[Kaf 11] שופרי—ŠWPRY: O. Occ / O. Cat. *sofre*, "sulphur"; cf. SHS 1:152–153, Gimel 11.

[Kaf 15] מירקא—MYRQ', or קטאפוסיא—QṬ'PWSY': The first term MYRQ' may represent Lat. *myrice* / *mirica*, "tamarisk" (genus Tamarix L.) (NPRA 167; GGA 482). The second term is Late Lat., O. Occ., or O. Cat. *catapucia* for "spurge" (Euphorbia lathyris L.); cf. SHS 1:152–153, Qof 21. Neither of these synonyms, however, matches the meaning of the Arab. term, which is "marshmallow" (Althea officinalis L.).

[Kaf 16] ארגוה—'RGWH, or שינבא—ŠYNB': 'RGWH represents O. Occ. or O. Cat. *eruga*, "garden rocket" (Eruca vesicaria sativa Mill.) (DAO 1099; DCVB 10:816a) with a metathesis; cf. also IT 16.3, among others. In accordance with the Arab. term, the second synonym is O. Occ. *senebe* for "(black) mustard" (Brassica nigra Koch) (DAO 905); cf. also SHS 2, Alef 25 and Shin 13; IT 13.4, among others.

[Kaf 17] קאשיפשטולא—Q'ŠYPŠṬWL': Late Lat. *cas(s)ia fistula*, or the corresponding O. Occ. / O. Cat. loanword documented as *cassia fistola* / *cassie fistule* / *cacia fistula*, "Indian laburnum" (Cassia fistula L.) (MLWB 2:327; DAO 1174; DECLC 2:619a); cf. IT 20.2.

[Kaf 18] לויאמי—LWY'MY: The Romance term *levame*, "leaven," is documented in Mod. Provençal (FEW 5:267a); in O. Occ. *levam*, id. (FEW 5:266b) is attested.

[Lamed 1] פלנטאגי—PLNṬ'ǦY: O. Occ. or O. Cat. *planta(t)ge* / *plantagi* for "ribwort" (Plantago lanceolata L.); cf. SHS 1:290–291, Lamed 12.

[Lamed 2] לאקא—L'Q': Lat. or Romance (O. Occ. / O. Cat.) *lac(c)a*, "shellac," the resin secreted by the bug Kerria lacca Kerr.; cf. SHS 1:121–122, Alef 41; and IT 8.3.

[Lamed 3] לנגא בובינא—LNG' BWBYN': O. Occ. *linga bovina* / *lenga bovina*, or O. Cat. *lingua bovina* for "bugloss" (Anchusa officialis L.); cf. SHS 1:292, Lamed 15.

[Lamed 5] גימאש או מרגרידש או פורלש—GYM'Š or MRGRYDŠ or PWRLŠ: The first term GYM'Š represents the (accusative) plural of Lat., O. Occ., or O. Cat. *gemma*, "precious stone" (FEW 4:94a; DAO 307; DCVB 6:252a). The second term, MRGRYDŠ, is the plural of O. Occ. / O. Cat. *margarida*, O. Occ. *marguerita*, "pearl" (FEW 6.1:323b; DCVB 7:244a; DECLC 5:487a–b). Finally, PWRLŠ transcribes the plural of O. Occ. / O. Cat. *perla* (RL 3:521a; DAO 307; DCVB 8:478b–479a). The letter waw is misspelled for Yod. All terms feature also in SHS-2, Gimel 9, Mem 17.

[Lamed 6] שרפנטינא—ŠRPNṬYN': The O. Occ. term (*herba*) *serpentina* designates plants of the genus Arum L. (DAO 969; FEW 11:521a).

[Lamed 7] לנגא אויש—LNG' 'WYŠ: The term is a Romance–Lat. *blend: linga/ lenga avis*, from Latin *lingua avis* designating the "ash" (Fraxinus excelsior L.); cf. SHS 1:286–287, Lamed 3.

[Mem 2] מוו—MWW: M. Lat. *meu* (FEW 6.2:64b) or O. Cat. *mèu* (DCVB 7:407b) for "spingel" (Meum athamanticum Jacq.); SHS 2, Mem 18.

[Mem 3] משתיק—MŠTYQ: Lat. *mastix*, O. Occ. / O. Cat *mastec(h)*, or O.Occ. *mastic* for "resin of the mastic tree" (Pistacia lentiscus L.); cf. SHS 1:336–337, Nun 2; IT 8.3, inter alia.

[Mem 4] בדליום גימיניס—BDLYWM GYMYNYS: Lat. *bdellium*, "resin of the plant Commiphora" (Commiphora mukul Engl.) (GGA 369; NPRA 34). The second element is probably specified by popular Lat. **Ieminis*, "from Yemen" (cf. ThLL 2:458 *Iemini*).

[Mem 5] פאירי איננס פיל—P'YRY 'YNNS PYL: O. Occ. **peire enans fil(h)*, or O. Cat. **paire enans fill*, literally "father before son." In SHS 1:104–105, Alef 18, the Romance term (P'YYRY 'YNY'S PYL, Ms O) is identified with the same Arab. and Hebr. terms (the Hebr. expression is probably an ad-hoc translation of the Romance term) and additionally with Lat. *oculus consulis*, "water mint" (Menta aquatica L.) and M. Lat. **antipatre*, which probably was the loan basis for our Romance term and for which different meanings can be found (e.g., Anthemis tinctoria L., Potentilla erecta Raeusch., Bellis perennis L.).

[Mem 6] דליום אינדיאני—DLYWM 'YNDY'NY: The first element of the compound term is Lat. *bdellium* (cf. entry [Mem 4] above); the second element belongs to the Lat. adjective *Indianum*, "Indian" (GH 2:191); the ending seems to be misspelled or is due to a confusion with O. Occ. *indi*, id.; for *indi* see SHS 1:96.

[Mem 7] מומיא—MWMY': O. Occ. *momia* (FEW 19:130b) or O. Cat. *momia / mumia* (DCVB 7:649b; DECLC 5:768a); it designates substances used for embalming (DECLC loc. cit.) and was also used to denote parts of mummies that were used in medicine (cf. DCVB loc. cit.). Cf. SHS 2, Mem 19.

[Mem 8] קטפוסיא מנור או קאקמיא—QṬPWSY' MNWR or Q'QMY': The first term represents Late Lat. *catapucia minor*, Ricinus communis (AdV 572). In AdV, it is identified with Arab. *ḥabb al-ḫirwaʿ* with the same meaning. Cf. also SHS 1:460, Qof 21, where the simplex Q'ṬPWSY' is interpreted as Late Lat., O. Occ., or O. Cat. *catapucia*, "spurge" (Euphorbis Lathyris; cf. also SHS 2, Qof 27: Q'ṬPWSY' MYNWR and Qof 24: Q'ṬPWSY' MGWR, *catapucia major*). The second term Q'QMY' seems to be related to Lat. *cacare*, "to shit": the FEW (2:18a) mentions several names of plants that cause diarrhea derived from *cacare*, although none of them matches the word found here (**cacamia*?).

[Mem 10] סילידוניאה מנור—SYLYDWNY'H MNWR: M. Lat. *c(h)elidonia minor*, "lesser celandine" (Ranunculus ficaria L.); cf. NPRA (62). For the M. Lat. simplex *celidonia*, cf. Sin (93, no. 80); and GGA (388). Cf. also the loanwords O. Occ. *selidonia* / *celidonia* (DAO 1138; FEW 2:634a) and O. Cat. *celidònia* (DCVB 3:100a); cf. IT 22.4.

[Mem 12] לוריולה—LWRYWLH: Lat. or O. Occ. *laureola*, which designates plants whose leaves have more or less the shape of those of the laurel; cf. SHS 1:103, Alef 16.

[Mem 13] מירא—MYR': Lat. *myrrha*, or O. Occ. / O. Cat. *mi(r)ra* for the aromatic resin "myrrh"; cf. SHS 1:307, Mem 8.

[Mem 14] אישטאפיזקרא או קפאפורגא—'YŠṬ'PYZQR' or QP'PWRG': The first term represents O. Occ. *estafizagra*, "stavesacre; lice-bane" (Delphinium staphisagria L.) (DAO 995). In O. Cat., only variants with the ending *-ia* are documented (*estafisàgria*, DCVB 5:502b); cf. IT 18.7. The second term, QP'PWRG', is probably a non-documented Romance variant **capapurga*, id., a loan translation of M. Lat. *caputpurgium* (FEW 9:614b, n. 3); also cf. M. Fr. *purge-chief*, id. (FEW 9:612b).

[Mem 15] ליטרג—LYṬRG: O. Occ. or O. Cat. *litargi* or *litarge* for "lead oxide"; cf. SHS 1:305–306, Mem 6.

[Mem 18] פירא קרמיטא—PYR' QRMYṬ': The compound represents O. Occ. / O. Cat. **peira caramida*, "magnetic stone." In SHS 1:312–313, Mem 18, we find the Lat.(–Romance) compound *lapis caramida* (Lat. *lapis*, "stone," and Late Lat. or Romance *caramida*, "magnetic stone"). For Romance intervocalic *-d-* transcribed by Hebrew Ṭ, see SHS 1:50–51. The term here is a Romance loan translation of Lat. *lapis magnes*, id. (GH 2:765). For O. Occ. *peira* / O. Cat. *pe(i)ra*, "stone," cf. FEW (8:313b); DAO (281); DCVB (8:442a).

[Nun 2] שלניטרי—ŠLNYṬRY: O. Occ. or O. Cat. *salnitre* or Lat. *sal nitri*, "natural soda, potassium nitrate"; cf. SHS 1:133, Bet 5.

[Nun 4] שלמוניאק—ŠLMWNY'Q: Romance **salmoniac* / **sal amoniac* for "gum ammoniac," a kind of gum resin used in medicine for making plasters. Usually, the Romance variants show an epenthetic *-r-*, as in O. Occ. *sal armoniac* or O. Cat. *armoniac(h)* (from Lat. *sal ammoniacus*). In the FEW (24:459a), a M. Fr. variant without *-r-*, *sel ammoniac*, is documented, as well as in Ibn Tibbon's translation, 'MWNY'Q, which is probably O. Occ. (IT 15.9, inter alia). Cf. SHS 1:335–336, Nun 1.

[Nun 5] אמאוש—'M'WŠ: Late Lat., O. Occ., O. Cat., or O. Sp. *ameos* for "a kind of umbellifer," probably "Bishop's weed" (Ammi visnaga L.); cf. SHS 1:337, Nun 3.

[Nun 6] אמידום—'MYDWM: Lat. *amidum* for "wheat flour"; cf. SHS 1:217, Ḥet 14.

[Nun 7] פוג גרדישג—PWG GRDYŠG: Romance, most probably O. Occ., **foc grezesc* for "Greek fire," an incendiary weapon used in ancient and medieval times, particularly in naval battles. The term is documented as O. Occ. *foc gresle*, id. (FEW 4:209a) / O. Cat. *foc grec*, id. (DCVB 5:935b). The O. Occ. adjective *grezesc*, "Greek," also appears in the variant GRDYŠQ (inter alia) in IT 18.5. (cf. also WfP 311). Cf. SHS 1:49–50 for Romance [z] represented by Dalet and the final voiceless consonant [k] transcribed by Gimel.

[Samekh 1] ארמודקטיל—'RMWDQṬYL (Ms. ב): O. Occ. or O. Cat. *(h)ermodactil*; for O. Occ., the DAO (1120) gives the meaning Iris tuberosa L., whereas the DCVB (6:517b) indicates the meaning Colchicum autumnale L. for the O. Cat. word, in accordance with the Arab. synonym. Cf. SHS 2, He 2. The reading 'RMWDYNṬYLY (Ms. א) seems to be misspelled.

[Samekh 2] פיש דשייט—PYŠ DŠYYṬ: Romance **peix de saget*. The term is documented in O. Cat. as *pe(i)x saget* (DCVB 8:383a) and in O. Sp. as *pez saget* (DETEMA 2:1218c), literally "arrow fish," for "a kind of fish used as aphrodisiac." The identification of Lat. *piscis sagitta* with *stincus* (a variant of *scincus*), meaning "skink" (Scincus officinalis, possibly Chalcides chalcides, or Chalcides ocellatus), is given in Sin (145,25, inter alia). Cf. also HebMedSyn 189 f., where the vernacular PYŠŠ'YYṬ (O. Cat. *peix saget*?) is identified with the same Arab. word as the one given in the *Sefer Almansur*. The term **peix de saget* rather seems to be O. Cat. than O. Occ., since "arrow" is *sa(g)eta* (FEW 11:58a; LR 5:132b) in O. Occ., with preservation of the Lat. final vowel.

[Samekh 3] ריקליציאה—RYQLYṢY'H: O. Occ. *recales(s)ia* (also: *regalecia* / *regalis(s)ia*; cf. O. Cat. *regalícia* / *regalèssia* / *regalíssia*) for "licorice"; cf. SHS 1:522–523, Shin 519.

[Samekh 4] שיזליוס—ŠYZLYWS: M. Lat. *siseleos*, Laserpitium L. or Seseli tortuosum L. ("hartwort"); cf. also IT 18.5.

[Samekh 5] מאפיר—M'PYR: The term is possibly a corruption of סראפי (SR'PY), which figures as a variant in Ms. ב. It may represent O. Occ. or O. Cat. *serapi(n)* for "sagapenum," i.e., the gum resin of Ferula Scowitziana D.C. (DAO 568 *serapin*; FEW 11:669a id.; DCVB 9:853b serapí). Also cf. IT (10.5) for O. Cat. *sagapí*, id.

[Samekh 6] סומאקו—SWM'QW: The term corresponds to M. Lat. *sumacum* (which existed besides *sumac*).[10] O. Occ. / O. Cat. had variants without final vowel of the type *sumac(h)*. Cf. SHS 1:93–94, Alef 3.

[Samekh 7] אשקמוניאה—'ŠQMWNY'H: Romance (O. Occ. / O. Cat.) *escamonea*, "resin of the plant scammony" (Convolvulus scammonia L.) (FEW 11:276a;

10 Less probably it corresponds to Old Italo-Romance variants such as *sumaco* or *sommaco* (FEW 19:164b).

DCVB 5:202a). According to FEW (11:276b), the term was used in the Middle Ages to designate a purgative drug made of this plant, but only from the sixteenth century onwards to designate the plant itself.

[Samekh 8] שינא שאנה—ŠYN', Š'NH: The term appearing here twice with a different spelling is M. Lat., O. Occ., or O. Cat. *sene* (< Arab. *sanā'*) for Cassia officinalis (Rhynchosia senna var. angustifolia [A. Gray] Grear); cf. SHS 1:372, Samekh 39: Š'N'; and GGA 537. The transcriptions, however, are uncommon and may suggest variants like **sena* (ŠYN') or **sane* (Š'NH), which are, apart from It. *sen(n)a* (FEW 19:153b), not documented in the Romance sources we consulted.

[Samekh 11] שבשתאן—ŠBŠT'N: M. Lat. *sebesten* / *sebestin*, "fruit of the sebesten tree" (Cordia Myxa L.). The term is documented for the Romance languages only in modern times; cf. SHS 1:148, Gimel 3.

[Samekh 12] קלאשא—QL'Š': M. Lat. or Romance (O. Occ. / Cat.) *clas(s)a*; the term was used to designate different kinds of resins, e.g., of juniper (Juniperus communis L.) (GGA 166). In the analysis of the Romance terms in Ibn Tibbon's *Sefer Ẓedat ha-Derakhim*, it is stated that in Europe, the resin of the juniper was often used for purposes similar to those of the sandarach tree (Tetraclinis articulate Masters) or was confused with it (cf. IT 25.11).

[Samekh 13] סאפיריסוס—S'PYRYSWS: Lat. *cyparissus*, "cypress" (Cupressus sempervivens and Var.) (NPRA 84). The permutation of Yod and Alef is probably an error.

[Samekh 14] סיפרום אורטירגאנגלי—SYPRYM, 'WRṬYRG'NGLY: Both vernacular words are identified with the Arab. and Hebr. words for the "long galingale" (Cyperus longus). The first term is Lat. *cyperum* for "root of a type of rush" (Cyperus longus and Var.) (cf. SHS 1:374–375, Samekh 44). The second one is probably to be interpreted as 'W RṬYR G'NGLY, with 'W meaning "or." RṬYR G'NGLY may be corrupt for *razis* [*de*] *galengal*, "root of galingale" (cf. FEW 19:61b for *galengal*; DAO 395 for *razis*, "root").

[Samekh 15] קרנק—QRNQ: O. Occ. or O. Cat. *cranc(h)* for "crab"; cf. SHS 1:429, Ṣade 1.

[Samekh 16] אשפיק—'ŠPYQ: O.Occ. *espic* / *aspic* or O. Cat. *espic* for "spike lavender" (Lavandula latifolia Medik.) (DAO 1064; FEW 12:174a; DCVB 5:424b). Cf. also SHS 1:501–502, Shin 10 (*espicanardi* = Nardostachys Jatamansi).

[Samekh 17] קשיאה ליניא—QŠY'H LYNY': Late Latin, O. Occ., or O. Cat. *cassia lignea*, "Chinese cinnamon" (Cinnamomum cassia [L.] D. Don); cf. SHS 1:466, Qof 34.

[Samekh 18] מלאבטרום—ML'BṬRWM: Lat. *malabat(h)rum*, "leaves of different kinds of plants, e.g., of Cinnamomum tamala Nees et var." (NPRA 151 f.; GGA 472); cf. SHS 2, Mem 29.

[Ayin 1] וירגא פשטורא—WYRG' PŠṬWR': Romanized variant of M. Lat. *virga pastoris*, "knotgrass" (Polygonum aviculare L.) (GGA 567).

[Ayin 2] פליטרי—PLYṬRY: O. Occ. or O. Cat. *pelitre*, "pellitory; feverfew" (Anacyclus pyrethrum [L.] Link); cf. SHS 1:181–182, He 2.

[Ayin 3] סילידוניה פיקה—SYLYDWNYH PYQH, and סילידוניה גראנ⟨ד⟩א—SYLYDWNYH GR'N[D]': The first synonym is a Romance (O. Occ. / O. Cat.) term **celidonia* (*celdonia*, DAO 1138), "celandine," specified with an adjective, perhaps *pega(?)* or *fera*, both probably meaning "wild." For Lat. / Romance *celidonia*, cf. entry [Mem 10] above. The O. Occ. / O. Cat. adjective *pec* / *pega*, which properly means "foolish" (FEW 8:116a; LR 5:475b; DCVB 8:350a), possibly takes the meaning of "wild, uncultivated" here. Alternatively, PYQH may be misspelled for *fera* (fem.), "wild" (FEW 3:478a; DCVB 5:802b). The second term, SYLYDWNYH GR'N[D]', is a Romance compound **celidonia grande*, a loan translation of Lat. *chelidonia maior*, "greater celandine" (Chelidonium majus L.) (NPRA 62). For O. Occ. / O. Cat. *gran* / *grande*, "great," cf. RL 3:497b; and DCVB 6:371a. Cf. also IT 22.4 for simple Lat. *celidonia*, which is a translation of Arab. ('L)KRKRM, "curcuma," among others. Cf. also Lat. *chelidonia minor*, "lesser celandine" (Ranunculus ficaria L.), which is discussed above (entry [Mem 10]).

[Ayin 4] מברילה—MBRYLH: O. Occ. *maurel(h)a*, or *maurella* for "black nightshade" (Solanum nigrum L.); cf. SHS 1:379–380, Ayin 4.

[Ayin 6] גנברי—GNBRY: O. Occ. and O. Cat. *ginebre* is "juniper" (Juniperus communis L.); cf. SHS 1:100, Alef 12.

[Ayin 7] טרבנטינא—ṬRBNṬYN': M. Lat. *ter(e)binthina*, O. Occ. *ter(r)ebentina* / *terbentina* / *trebentina*, or Cat. *terebentina* for "resin of pine trees; resin of Pistachia terebinthus L."; cf. SHS 1:299–300, Lamed 29.

[Ayin 8] שפראן אורטואל—ŠPR'N 'RṬW'L: The compound term is probably related to the O. Occ. term **safran ortola* ("garden safflower"), which figures in SHS 1:209, Ḥet 1, as ŠPR'N 'WRṬWL'N (Ms P). *Ortola(n)* is the O. Occ. / O. Cat. term for "gardener" (cf. loc. cit.).

[Ayin 9] רומזי—RWMZY: O. Occ. *romeze* for "common brumble" (Rubus fructicosus L.); cf. SHS 1:467, Qof 35.

[Ayin 10] ארנש—'RNŠ: Plural of O. Occ. or O. Cat. *arn* with the meaning "thorny bush, Christ's thorn" (Paliurus australis); cf. SHS 1:124, Alef 44.

[Pe 1] פברי—PBRY: Rom. (O. Occ. or O. Cat.) *pebre*, "pepper" (Piper nigrum); cf. SHS 1:415, Pe 25.

[Pe 2] ולריאנה—WLRY'NH: M. Lat *valeriana*, "valerian" (Valeriana officinalis L.; Valeriana phu L.) (cf. FEW 14,135ab). The M. Lat. term was also used as loan word in the Romance languages (for O. Occ. and O. Cat. see RL 5:465b; DCVB 10:652a); cf. SHS 2, Waw 6.

[Pe 3] איפורבי—'YPWRBY: The term appears in the same spelling in IT 18.7, where it is interpreted as O. Occ. *eforbi*, a variant of the more common *euforbi*, "spurge" (Euphorbia L.); (DAO 1140). For O. Cat., only variants with an initial diphthong (*eu-*) are documented.

[Pe 4] ליסיאום—LYSY'WM: Cf. entry [Ḥet 10].

[Pe 5] פראשיום—PR'ŠYWM: Late Lat. *prasium*, "horehound" (Marrubium vulgare L.); cf. SHS 1:285, Lamed 1.

[Pe 6] פאווינה—P'WWYNH: O. Occ. *peonia* or Lat. *paeonia*, "peony" (Paeonia L.). In Cat., this word does not appear before the fifteenth century; cf. SHS 1:520–521, Shin 46.

[Pe 8] אוילאנא אינדיגא—'WYL'NH 'YNDYG': O. Occ. *avelana* **indiga* or **endega*, an Occitanized form of Late Lat. *abellana indica*; the adjective 'YNDYG' shows the result of Western Romance lenition. The meaning is "areca nut," fruit of the Areca catechu L., according to the Arabic synonym, which also appears in SHS 1:300, Lamed 30.

[Pe 9] זינושקא שטוש—ZYNWŠQ' ŠṬWŠ: The vernacular term is wrongly separated into words: if we read ZYNWŠ Q'ŠṬWŠ and assume that the first letter of the first word is corrupt, we can interpret the compound term as Lat. *agnus castus*, "chaste tree" (Vitex agnus castus L.); cf. SHS 1:114–115, Alef 30, Ms O. This interpretation is also suggested by the meaning of the Arab. synonym.

[Pe 10] רוביה—RWBYH: Lat. *rubia*, "dyer's madder" (Rubia tinctorum L.) (NPRA 220). The phytonym is documented in O. Occ. as *roia* or *rubi*, inter alia (DAO 946, FEW 10:537a). Our variant rather resembles the Cat. variant *rubia*, which, in texts in Latin script, is documented only since the seventeenth century (cf. DCVB 9:605b).

[Pe 12] פוליג—PWLYG: O. Occ. *pol(i)eg* / *pul(i)eg*, or O. Cat. *polig* (but note that in O. Cat. the diminutive *poliol* or similar forms seem to have been more frequent) for "a kind of mint"; cf. SHS 1:258–259, Yod 17.

[Pe 14] בידיליה—BYDYLYH: The Romance term is probably Cat. *vidiella* / *vediella*, a species of "clematis" (DCECH 5:804ab; DCVB 10:795b–796a). Most of the Occitan variants listed in FEW (14:553ab) are quite different from ours, but some of the modern Occitan dialect forms mentioned there suggest that an O. Occ. **bidelha* or **bedilha* may have existed. Cf. SHS 2, Bet 22.

[Pe 16] יופארקי—YWP'RQY: Latin genitive singular of *hypericum*, i.e., *hyperici*. The meaning is "St. John's wort" (Hypericum perforatum L.); cf. SHS 2, Alef 70.

[Ṣade 1] אילוואי—'YLWW'Y: M. Lat. *aloe* meaning, among others, Aloe vera L., Aquilaria L., or its juice. The Lat. word was also used in various Romance languages: in O. Occ. and O. Cat., we find *aloe(n)*; cf. SHS 1:110, Alef 23.

[Ṣade 2] גומא—GWM': M. Lat. *gumma* or O. Occ. and O. Cat. *goma*, "gum"; cf. SHS 1:451–452, Qof 7.

[Ṣade 3] גומא ארביקא—GWM' 'RBYQ': M. Lat. *gumma arabica* or Romance (O. Occ./O. Cat.) *goma arabica* for "gum arabic" (cf. SHS 1:452, Qof 7).

[Ṣade 4] קוקליא—QWQLY': O. Occ. or O. Cat. *cauquilha* / *cauquila*, "shell"; cf. SHS 1:341–342, Nun 10.

[Qof 2] קראוי שלואיג—QR'WY ŠLW'YG: The term also appears in SHS 1:468, Qof 37, where it is interpreted as a non-documented O. Occ. or O. Cat. compound term **carvi salva(t)ge* for "wild, non-cultivated caraway."

[Qof 3] סינטוריא—SYNṬWRY': The Lat. term *centaurea*, "centaurea" (Centaurea erythrae) (NPRA 55; GGA 389), was also used in O. Occ. (*centauria* / *centaurea*, DAO 1146) and O. Cat. (*centaurea*, DCVB 3:111b); cf. SHS 2, Alef 83.

[Qof 5] קרדמומי—QRDMWMY: Genitive of Lat. *cardamomum* or O. Occ. *cardamomi*, "(seeds of the) green cardamom" (Elettaria cardamomum Maton.) (NPRA 49; FEW 2:365a; DAO 1175). In O. Cat., the plant was named *cardamom* / *cardamomia* / *cardimoni* (DCVB 2:1027b).

[Qof 6] סיטרולי או גלבנום—SYṬRWLY or GLBNWM: SYṬRWLY is probably O. Occ. *citruli*, "cucurbita" (Cucurbita L.) (DAO 860,4–2). The second term, GLBNWM, is Lat. *galbanum* "galbanum" (gum resin of Ferula galbaniflua) (GGA 433; GH 1:2896), in accordance with the meaning of the Arab. synonym. Cf. also SHS 2, Gimel 15.

[Qof 12] גראנא דשאפראן—GR'N' DŠ'PR'N: The compound term is O. Occ. *grana de safran*, "grains of safflower" (Crocus sativus L.); cf. O. Occ. *safran*, "safflower" (RL 5:131a), and O. Occ. *grana*, "grain; seed" (RL 2:495b). The O. Cat. variants for "safran" show the loss of final *-n* (*safrà*, DECLC 7:582b). Cf. also SHS 1:150, Gimel 5; and 209, Ḥet 1; SHS 2, Qof 13.

[Qof 17] אישפלטום היהודי גנאגום—'YŠPLṬWM HYHWDY GN'GWM(?): The first term 'YŠPLṬWM HYHWDY is a mixed Lat.–Hebr. compound; the first element is Lat. *aspaltum*, "asphalt, bitumen" (MLWB 1:1042); the second one is Hebr. HYHWDY, "of the Jews." The term is documented in the *Alphita* as *bitumen judaicum*, a synonym of *aspaltum* (GGA 361); cf. also *aspaltum Iudaicum* (ThLL 2:829). Cf. SHS 2, Alef 43. The second term GN'GWM(?) could not be identified.

[Qof 19] קלאמוש ארומאטיגא—QL'MWŠ 'RWM'ṬYG': The term is related to Lat. *calamus aromaticus*, "perfumed reed; false sweet flag" (Acorus calamus L.), which was also used in Romance medico-botanical texts (cf. SHS 1:450, Qof 5). The O. Occ. adjective *aromatic*, "aromatic" (FEW 25:293a), appears here in its feminine form *aromatica*, contrary to the gender of the noun.

[Resh 1] קוברי ארש או פרט לטי' אאישאו שיתום—QWBRY 'RŠ or PRṬ, in Latin ''YŠ'W ŠYTWM: The first term is the O. Occ. compound *coure/covre ars*, "burned copper"; cf. SHS 1:351, Nun 29. PRṬ may be an incomplete transcription of O. Occ. *perites*, "inflammable metallic sulfure" (DAO 344, 6–1), or of Lat. *pyrites, -ae*, "flintstone" (GH 2:2106); for Cat., there is no medieval documentation. Alternatively, PRṬ could be interpreted as O. Occ. / O. Cat. *ferret*, "little piece of iron," or "(medical) instrument of iron; poker" (FEW 3:471a; DCVB 5:825b). The third synonym ''YŠ'W ŠYTWM is Lat. *aes ustum*, "burnt copper" (GGA 379, *es ustum*), which is also identified with *coure ars* in SHS 2, Alef 80.

[Resh 2] ראיש ברברש—R'YŠ BRBRŠ: Non-documented masculine variant of Lat. *reubarbarum / reobarbarum*, "rhubarb" (Rheum ribes L.) (cf. SHS 1:538, Tav 19), i.e., **r(h)eus barbarus*. As in SHS 1 (loc. cit.), the Hebrew spelling shows a -Y- in the first word, which might be erroneous for a -W- (representing the vowel /u/ or /o/). But note that in O. Occ., variants like *reybarby / reibarbi* (frozen genitive forms) are documented (DAO 912), which might have influenced the transcription.

[Resh 3] דאגה דפין—D'GH DPYN: According to the Arab. and Hebr. synonyms, the Romance term should designate the "resin of the pine tree." While the second element (D)PYN can easily be interpreted as O. Occ. / O. Cat. *(de) pin*, "(of) pine tree" (FEW 8:548a; DCVB 8:547a; note that in Cat., the variant *pi* without final *-n* is more frequent), the first element presents difficulties. The usual O. Occ. / O. Cat. word for "resin" is *resina* (FEW 10:299a; DCVB 9:410a; cf. also DAO 562), which is obviously not transcribed here. Perhaps we should assume an influence of Lat. *sagapenum*, "resin of the Ferula communis L." (**saga de pin*?) (for *sagapenum* see GGA 528; NPRA 223; cf. also SGPY for O. Cat. **sagapí*, id., in IT 10.5).

[Resh 4] פנוייל—PNWYYL: O. Occ. *fenol(h)* (also spelled *fenoil(h) / fenoyl / fenoil(l)*), or O. Cat. *fenoll / fenoyl* for "fennel" (Foeniculum officinale L.); cf. SHS 1:504, Shin 13.

[Resh 5] סירנא—SYRN': The vernacular term is probably a metathetic variant of O. Occ. *senre* (variant of *cendre*) or of O. Cat. *cenra* (variant of *cendra*), "ashes" (FEW 2:684a; DCVB 3:106b)., which matches the meaning of the Arab. and Hebr. synonyms.

[Shin 3] שן שלמון—ŠN ŠLMWN: The Romance term also appears in SHS 2, Samekh 21, in the spelling Š'N ŠLMWN (Mss PV). It is identified there, among others, with SQQWL (Mss PO), i.e., Lat. *secacul*, "a kind of parsnip" (Malabaila secacul [Mill.] Boiss.) (GGA 536),[11] and with ŠGYLWM ŠLMWNYŠ (Mss PO)

11 In the *Alphita* it is said, "secacul, id est, yringos" (S 147), but it was already stated in

i.e., *sigillum Salomonis*, "Solomon's seal" (Polygonatum odoratum [Mill.] Druce or Polygonatum officinale All.) (GGA 540). The term ŠN ŠLMWN seems to be an O. Occ. compound term **sen*(*h*) [*de*] *Salomon*, O. Occ. *sen*(*h*) meaning "sign; seal" (< Lat. *signum*, "sign"; cf. FEW 11:605a) or an analogous O. Cat. **seny* [*de*] *Salomo*(*n*) (*for seny*, see DCVB 9:839a). Thus, it is a calque of the Latin *sigillum Salomonis* mentioned above. A similar version can be found in M. Fr. *signet de Salomon*, Polygonatum Mill. (FEW 11:608a).

[Shin 5] גוליום—GWLYWM: Lat. *jolium* for "darnel grass" (Lolium temulentum L.); cf. SHS 1:531–532, Tav 6.

[Shin 6] קבשיא—QBŠY': The M. Lat. term *capsia*, "peppergrass" (Lepidium latifolium L.), figures in the same peculiar spelling with -B- in SHS 1:399–400, Ayin 39, and in IT 18.4. In the SHS 1 (loc. cit.), it is also identified with Arab. *šīṭarağ*.

[Shin 7] אישולא או טיטמאל—'YŠWL' or ṬYṬM'L: The first term is M. Lat. *esula* for "spurge" (Euphorbia L.) (FEW 21:191b); the second one is O. Cat. / O. Occ. *titimal*, which has the same meaning (cf. SHS 1:509, Shin 22). The same synonymy of the two phytonyms appears in the *Alphita* (T7, see GGA 304).

[Shin 8] לאפיש אמאטיטש—L'PYŠ 'M'ṬYṬŠ: Lat. *lapis haematites*, "the stone haematite" (cf. GH 2:560 for *lapis*; GH 1:3003 for *haematites*). In Lat., it was common to add *lapis* to the name of the stone (cf. the designations of several stones in the *Alphita*, see GGA 460 ff.).[12]

[Shin 9] אלום—'LWM: O. Occ. or O. Cat. *alum* for "alum"; cf. SHS 1:308, Mem 10.

[Shin 10] קלקא טריפה—QLQ' ṬRYPH: O. Occ. *calcatrepa*, "star-thistle" (Centaurea calpitrapa L.) (DAO 1146; FEW 2:65a); in O. Cat., the phytonym is not attested.

[Shin 11] פומוש טירא—PWMWŠ ṬYR': Late Lat., O. Occ., or O. Cat. *fumus terre*, *fumusterre*, "fumitory" (Fumaria officinalis L.); cf. SHS 1:522, Shin 50.

[Shin 12] שאוי—Š'WY: O. Occ. *seu* / *ceu* or O. Cat. *sèu*, "suet; sebum" (FEW 11:358b; DCVB 9:891a).

[Shin 14] רושילש—RWŠYLŠ: The same Arab., Hebr., and Romance phytonyms are used as synonyms in SHS 1:508, Shin 20. The Arab. and Hebr. plant names mean "anemone" (Anemone L.). This meaning is, in fact, attested for O. Cat. *rosella* (DCVB 9:580a–b), which appears here in the plural. Cf. also O. Occ. *rozel*(*l*)*a* / O. Cat. *rosella*, Papaver rhoeas, inter alia (DAO 1147; DCVB loc. cit.).

---

medieval times that two different plants were meant, i.e., *secacul* is a kind of parsnip, and *yringos* is "eryngo" (Eryngium campestre L.) (GGA loc. cit.).

12 Cf. also M 369; Berakhyah, *Sefer Ko'ah ha-Avanim* (eds. Bos and Zwink), pp. 93, 118–119 (no. 9): Angl.-Nor. **ematis* for *ematite*.

[Shin 15] גיט—GYṬ: Lat. *git* for "black cumin" (Nigella sativa L.); the name was also used in O. Occ. and O. Cat. medico-botanical texts; cf. SHS 1:457, Qof 17; and IT 16.2.

[Tav 3] תרביד—TRBYD: Romance or M. Lat. Arabism derived from the Arab. term featuring here, i.e., M. Lat. *turbith, turpeth* (*Operculina turpethum*) (GGA 563) or O. Occ./ O. Cat. *turbit / torbit*, id. (FEW 19:190a–b; DCVB 10:580a). Cf. SHS 1:50 for the Romance voiceless consonant [-t] transcribed by Dalet.

[Tav 4] מאנה—M'NH: O. Occ. or O. Cat. *man(n)a*, "kind of sugary extract of some plants (especially of the manna ash, Fraxinus ornus L.), used in medicine" (FEW 6.1:232a–233b; DAO 572, DCVB 7:206b); cf. SHS 2, Mem 21.

[Tav 5] תמראינדי—TMR'YNDY: O. Occ. / O. Cat. *tamarindi* for "fruit of the Tamarindus indica L." (FEW 19:180b; RPA 516; DCVB 10:125b); cf. IT 15.3, inter alia.

[Tav 6] טאפסיא—Ṭ'PSY': Lat. / O. Cat. *thapsia* or O. Occ. *tapsie*, "false fennel" (Thapsia garganica L.); cf. SHS 1:202–203, Zayin 10.

[Tav 7] אגורשטש אגרם—'GWRŠṬŠ 'GRM: The first synonym 'GWRŠṬŠ corresponds to a metathetic variant of Graeco–Lat. *agrostis* (f), "couch grass" (Cynodon dactylon Pers.) (NPRA 8; GH 1:280). The second one, 'GRM, is O. Cat. *agram*, id. (DCVB 6:367b). In SHS 1:219–220, Ḥet 17, Arab. *ṯīl* and Hebr. ḤṢB, id., are identified with O. Occ. / O. Cat. *gram*, id.

Indexes

Terms in Hebrew Characters (Hebrew, Arabic, Romance, and Latin)

English

Romance and Latin (as Interpreted from the Hebrew Forms)

vetriol / vitriol Zayin 5
vidiella. *See* bidalhe
virga pastoris Ayin 1
visc(h) Dalet 3
vitriol. *See* vetriol
*viva corvina Ḥet 4
vomita Gimel 1

Non-identified (Romance or Latin?) Terms

'NPSQ He 5
GN'GWM Qof 17
Ḥ('?)RYBBR' Gimel 12

ysop. *See* isop
ys(s)opus. *See* (h)yssopus

*zingebre Zayin 1

Printed in the United States
By Bookmasters